"Finally! A book that eloquently but concisely explains how certain dietary modifications can actually trigger your body's natural ability to activate your own coveted stem cells based on sound, scientific evidence. With a fantastic explanation of the various types of stem cells, Dr. Elia, gives you solid facts about how to optimize your stem cells, slow down your clock, improve your gut and immune health, and feel fantastic! You'll love reading about exactly what foods and dietary supplements to include and what to remove. And with her super easy-to-follow guidelines, you'll experience the benefits of stem cell activation right away!"

—Dr. Sheila Dean, DSc, RDN, LDN, IFMCP

Cofounder of the Integrative and Functional Nutrition Academy; adjunct professor at the University of Tampa and University of South Florida, Morsani College of Medicine

"In *Stem Cell Activation Diet*, Dr. Elia uses a conversational tone to dive into our way of living and to encourage us to leap into the changes that will make us feel better quickly and sustain us in health. She engages us in the physiology, science, and solutions. She provides comprehensive, practical, and specific recommendations for improving your lifestyle to engage your vitality. Although targeted to consumers, this book could easily be used as a textbook."

—Liz Lipski, PhD, CNS, BCHN, IFMCP, LDN

Professor at Maryland University of Integrative Health, author of *Digestive Wellness*, and founder of the Innovative Healing Academy

T0088098

"A diet book informed by science and written by a credible nutrition expert whose personal health journey lead her to meticulously researching the potential of stem cells. Packed with nutritional strategies to tap into the regenerative power of using both food and fasting as medicine!"

—Kathie Madonna Swift, MS, RDN, LDN, FAND,
author of *The Swift Diet*

THE
STEM CELL
ACTIVATION DIET

Your COMPLETE NUTRITIONAL GUIDE
to Fight Disease, Support Brain Health,
and Slow the Effects of Aging

DANA ELIA
DCN-C, MS, RDN, LDN, FAND

ULYSSES PRESS

Published in the United States by:
ULYSSES PRESS
P.O. Box 3440
Berkeley, CA 94703
www.ulyssespress.com

ISBN: 978-1-64604-011-7
Library of Congress Control Number: 2019951365

Printed in the United States by Kingery Printing Company
10 9 8 7 6 5 4 3 2 1

Acquisitions editor: Bridget Thoreson
Managing editor: Claire Chun
Project editor: Renee Rutledge
Editor: Barbara Schultz
Index: S4Carlisle
Front cover design: David Hastings
Artwork: all from shutterstock.com—cells (cover/chapter graphics) © Nixx
    Photography; cover fruits and vegetables © StudioPhotoDFlorez; page 96
    © GraphicsRF
Interior design: Jake Flaherty

NOTE TO READERS: This book has been written and published strictly for informational and educational purposes only. It is not intended to serve as medical advice or to be any form of medical treatment. You should always consult your physician before altering or changing any aspect of your medical treatment and/or undertaking a diet regimen, including the guidelines as described in this book. Do not stop or change any prescription medications without the guidance and advice of your physician. Any use of the information in this book is made on the reader's good judgment after consulting with his or her physician and is the reader's sole responsibility. This book is not intended to diagnose or treat any medical condition and is not a substitute for a physician. This book is independently authored and published and no sponsorship or endorsement of this book by, and no affiliation with, any trademarked brands or other products mentioned within is claimed or suggested. All trademarks that appear in ingredient lists and elsewhere in this book belong to their respective owners and are used here for informational purposes only. The author and publisher encourage readers to patronize the quality brands mentioned in this book.

*To my husband, James, who has been my rock,
constant cheerleader, and the perfect partner
to journey through this life with me.*

*To all those who seek to tap into the body's natural ability
to right itself when given the proper, yet basic tools.*

*May this book and my story serve as an inspiration
to follow your instincts and never cease to
be an advocate for your own health.*

CONTENTS

Chapter 9

DISCUSSIONS WITH THE EXPERTS 143

FINAL THOUGHTS.. 155

BIBLIOGRAPHY 157

INDEX.. 163

ACKNOWLEDGMENTS 171

ABOUT THE AUTHOR 172

INTRODUCTION

Welcome, and I look forward to providing you with some tools and resources to help you along your wellness journey. Some background on me, I've been a registered dietitian nutritionist (RDN) since 1996, having completed both my bachelor of science in dietetics and dietetic internship through Montclair State University. I have a master's in health sciences with a concentration in integrative health and wellness from Rutgers University, and am in the final phase of finishing my doctorate in clinical functional nutrition (DCN) at Maryland University of Integrative Health, with an expected completion date of April 2020. I feel fortunate to have worked in numerous areas of dietetics besides my private practice: inpatient, critical care, chief clinical dietitian, and home infusion. However, I've done some degree of private practice/consulting throughout my career. Today, I own a successful integrative and functional nutrition-based practice in Lancaster, and I teach an undergraduate Nutrition for Life course at the Pennsylvania College of Health Sciences.

Why Functional Nutrition?

I essentially grew up in an internist's office, as my mother was the office manager, and I originally thought I would go into medicine. I had my mind set on becoming a surgeon; even my earliest diaries record my dreams of a career in medicine. However, my own childhood and teenage health issues led me to nutrition and especially to my interest in the more integrative side, or complementary and alternative medicine, as we called it back then. Many of us practicing in the integrative and functional arena came to it because of our own personal health crises. I have dealt with my own health concerns and can attest to the power that food has to be medicine; it helps to make me a better clinician.

When applying key principles of functional nutrition to my own timeline, it's easy for me to see how my own health struggles came about. In fact, when teaching students or speaking to other clinicians, I often joke that my childhood was the perfect setup for a functional medicine case study. To help illustrate this, I'll share some of my personal history with you. My mother took the fertility drug Clomid to conceive, and she was most likely a gestational diabetic while pregnant with me, but no specific testing was done to her recollection. While I was in the womb, my mother developed appendicitis and had surgery during the eighth month of pregnancy, thereby exposing me to anesthesia, pain medications, and antibiotics in utero. I was born via cesarean section and not breastfed, as not only had my mother developed mastitis but also in the early 1970s it was common practice to discourage breastfeeding after a C-section due to the notion that breastfeeding would put too much pressure on the incision site.

As an infant, I was given soy-based formula due to having a "sensitive stomach." Essentially, I had been struggling with IBS issues from birth. I can even recall having bouts of insomnia from early childhood. Though I always looked forward to a good sleepover party, secretly I knew I would most likely be spending the night staring at the ceiling, unable to fall asleep in unfamiliar surroundings. From pre-kindergarten to second grade, there were numerous ear and throat infections; I spent more time on the "pink bubble gum" medicine (aka amoxicillin) than off of it. I was a frequent flyer at the pediatrician's office. I can still vividly remember the antiseptic smell, the steps down to the lab where the nurse would swab my throat and then a petri dish, and then the huge bubbles Dr. Flood would make with his soapy hands to help ease my fears.

In second grade, I was diagnosed with juvenile rheumatoid arthritis, and thus began the downward spiral of drugs and health issues all through elementary school, high school, and even into college. I was given various rounds of corticosteroids, high doses of aspirin, nonsteroidal anti-inflammatory drugs (NSAIDs), and eventually, Plaquenil and weekly methotrexate injections. By the time I was in college, my rheumatologist had added hypothyroidism, fibromyalgia, and systemic lupus erythematosus to my diagnosis list. Over the years, I experienced rapid changes in my vision, developed thyroid issues, continued to struggle with chronic irritable bowel syndrome with constipation (in my younger years I was often given mineral oil at bedtime), and battled with my weight. I knew there had to be a better way to manage my health than what I had experienced through traditional Western medicine.

My decision to study nutrition and dietetics instead of medicine was fueled by my quest to help heal my own body, manage my ballooning weight, and find success where conventional therapies had failed me. Throughout my journey, I've seen the direct correlation that infections, stress, diet and exercise changes, and environmental exposures had on my symptoms and RA flares. Things were going smoothly until May 2013, when I was diagnosed with a rare sarcoma in my left abdominal wall, close to where my weekly methotrexate injections were given. I credit a functional nutrition approach to keeping me from needing any medications for my autoimmune issues for close to twenty years now, as well as helping me to maintain a healthy weight.

Why My Interest in Stem Cells?

I've spent my entire career reading the research and following the ever-evolving body of literature on various styles of diets and how they impact health outcomes. One area of focus that caught and held my attention was the area of fasting and fasting-mimicking diets. Beginning in 2016, I made some targeted changes to my chosen type of diet, supplement regimen, and style of workouts, with significant results. For example, I began toying around with time-restricted feeding (we'll get into more details later on various fasting approaches) and followed a 14:10 fasting regimen, meaning I would fast for fourteen hours and then consume my daily meals within a ten-hour window. Presently, I follow a 16:8 regimen. Within the first few days, my energy improved and I was sleeping better. For years, I have been in the habit of tracking my food intake and activity. These logs were useful in showing that while my calories, macronutrient intake, and caloric expenditure through activity were relatively unchanged, after the first few weeks, I began to lose weight. Honestly, I was more interested in the overall health benefits of fasting, but I didn't mind the added benefit of the weight loss.

After wearing the same size clothing for over fifteen years, I now needed a new wardrobe, having dropped two sizes. Plus, in my HIIT workouts, I noticed my strength and endurance was markedly improved and progressing more. When I reevaluate those changes on my functional medicine timeline, it cements my belief in the level of impact these changes have made.

In the winter of 2017–18, my left elbow was causing me significant pain and impacting my workouts. In February 2018, I was told that I needed to have my left lateral epicondyle surgically repaired after the months of physical therapy (PT) and nutrition support hadn't provided enough improvement. When reviewing the MRI, my orthopedic surgeon commented that "no amount of diet or PT" would repair the tendon. Surgery was inevitable and scheduled. During the two weeks between the consult and surgery, I turned my attention to researching some nonsurgical options. I looked into stem cell injections. However, given the lack of research on stem cell injections for those of us with a history of rare cancers, I opted for the surgical route. Still, having already completed a few rounds of a fasting protocol, I opted to do another round of the protocol the week before surgery. Hindsight being 20/20, I wish there had been an opportunity to have a pre-fast and post-fast MRI done. The surgery went well and in the recovery room, my surgeon seemed a bit stumped. He explained how my tendon still needed to be repaired, but what he couldn't explain was how different the tendon now looked two weeks after the MRI. I shared with him my fasting program details, the research behind it, and its impact on stem cell activation. I'll go into great detail later in this book about the different approaches to fasting and the specifics on the program I have used personally and in my practice.

The complexity of my own medical history has made me passionate about integrative and functional nutrition, and food as medicine. My wish is to see the day when all future dietitian nutritionists have a strong foundation in integrative and functional medical nutrition therapy. To help work toward this goal, I've been actively involved in the executive committee of Dietitians in Integrative and Functional Medicine since 2013 and am currently serving as Chair (2019–20).

I am living proof of the power of food. When the right diet and lifestyle choices are given priority in your life, your body possesses an innate ability to heal. In 25 years of practice, I have never recommended anything for a client that I have not researched and/or tried myself. I believe in our ability to harness the force within us and optimize our stem cells through our food choices. I hope that by the end of this book, you will be empowered, enlightened, and energized to tap into your own healing power.

Chapter 1

A CRASH COURSE ON STEM CELLS

Simply stated, stem cells are essential for the development and continued maintenance of all tissues and organs in the body. According to the National Institutes of Health (NIH), stem cells are "cells with the ability to divide for indefinite periods in culture and to give rise to specialized cells."[1] Your stem cells have been working for you since conception. We all originally *stem* from stem cells! However, out of the 37 billion cells in your body, stem cells account for only 0.002 percent! Consider them the main players in your body's maintenance crew, the ultimate raw material, each day working to generate, regenerate, and renew your body and your health. If your stem cells suddenly went on strike, death would occur within a week. These powerhouse workers regenerate the cells of your:

• small intestine every four to five days

• lungs and stomach every eight days

• skin every two weeks

---

1   National Institute of Health, "Stem Cell Information Home Page."

- blood cells every three to four months
- fat cells every eight years
- skeleton every ten years

Miracle Worker Cells

Three main features set stem cells apart from other types of cells in the body. The first feature is that they are unspecialized or undifferentiated cells. Cells that are classified as differentiated are cells that are specialized to perform a specific job duty in the body. By being undifferentiated cells, stem cells do not have one particular role; rather, they have the opportunity to have many. The second feature is they possess the ability to renew themselves by a process called cell division. This process can even occur after extended periods of time with no activity in the cell. The third feature of stem cells is that with the right conditions they can become specialized tissue, or organ-specific, cells. This process can occur both under biological conditions in the body or under experimental conditions in a lab.

Because of their unique qualities, stem cells hold enormous possibilities as an innovative therapeutic intervention. Stem cells possess the ability to differentiate or develop into many types of cells, and this ability makes them useful for the treatment of a variety of degenerative diseases. Stem cells have the power to repair, and the capacity for self-renewal, replenishment, and differentiation is the major characteristic that sets them apart from all other cells.

When not renewing themselves, these miracle worker cells answer the body's call and can change into more specialized cells such as blood cells, brain cells, heart muscle, or bone. For example, in the gut and bone marrow, stem cells divide on a regular basis in order to repair and replace worn-out or damaged tissues in those organs. In other organs, like the pancreas and the heart, the process only occurs under special conditions.

Where Do Stem Cells Come From?

I promise the rest of this chapter will be the most scientific part of the entire book, but I want to briefly explain the ways that scientific literature and textbooks discuss stem cells. There are four main categories of stem cells: embryonic, adult, fetal, and cord blood. Within these categories are numerous different types of cells. Below are the NIH's definitions of the two most commonly discussed categories of stem cells, embryonic and adult.[2]

1. **Embryonic stem cells** are primitive (undifferentiated) cells derived from a five-day preimplantation embryo that are capable of dividing without differentiating for a prolonged period in culture, and are known to develop into cells and tissues of the three primary germ layers. (Germ layers are the primary cell layers that are formed in the early stages of embryonic development. There are three layers: inner layer [endoderm], outer layer [ectoderm], and middle layer [mesoderm].)

2. **Somatic (adult) stem cells** are relatively rare undifferentiated cells found in many organs and differentiated tissues with a limited capacity for both self-renewal (in the laboratory) and differentiation. Such cells vary in their differentiation capacity, but it is usually limited to cell types in the organ of origin.

Some key differences between the two: Embryonic stem cells are retrieved from embryos that are four to six days old. These embryos are obtained from fertility clinics where they have been

---

2   National Institute of Health, "Stem Cell Information Home Page."

donated or were created with the intent to be used for research, so that stem cells could be harvested from them and used for therapeutic cloning. Therapeutic cloning is also referred to as somatic cell nuclear transfer (SCNT).

Depending on your age, you may remember Dolly, the first sheep cloned in 1997. Presently researchers in South Korea are the only scientists to have claimed success in the creation of human embryos by means of therapeutic cloning. These scientists have also claimed success in harvesting stem cells from these cloned embryos. In the United States SCNT is legal, but a moratorium on United States federal funding for SCNT issued in 2002 prohibits federal funding from being used for SCNT research. The main goal for the researchers using SCNT is not to produce children; it's to obtain embryonic stem cells that can then be harvested and made into cell-based therapies.

Adult stem cells are already designated for a certain organ or tissue. Some adult stem cells can be coaxed into or be reprogrammed into turning into a different type of specialized cell within the tissue type. For example, heart stem cells can give rise to a functional heart muscle cell, but it is still unclear whether they can give rise to all different cell types of the body. It's important to point out that the term *adult* when referring to adult stem cells is not meant to imply that they are only found in adults. They are found in children. Here the term *adult* is used to mean a stem cell being found in a developed organism.

During the 1980s, in mouse model experiments, scientists uncovered the means to obtain embryonic stem cells from mouse embryos. Fast-forward to the late 1990s, when that knowledge derived from mice models was applied to discover a method to draw stem cells from human embryos and grow those cells in a laboratory setting. These were the first human embryonic stem cells.

Human embryonic stem cell: A type of pluripotent stem cell (see definition below) that is derived from the inner cell mass of the blastocyst. (A blastocyst is the cluster of cells in the beginning stages of embryonic development. The inner cluster gives rise to the embryo and the outer layer of cells becomes the placenta and other supporting tissues needed for fetal development.)

Embryos used for fertility procedures, such as in-vitro fertilization, are donated with consent for the purpose of research. In 2006, scientists made another important discovery when determining the necessary specific conditions to return a specialized adult cell back to an unspecialized stem-cell-like state. This process of genetically "reprogramming" created a new type of stem cells, called induced pluripotent stem cells (iPSCs).

Induced pluripotent stem cells: Somatic (adult) cells reprogrammed to enter an embryonic, unspecialized stem cell–like state.

Important Terms

Potency: The stem cell's ability to differentiate into specialized cell types and be able to give rise to any mature cell.

Totipotent (or Omnipotent) Stem Cells: These cells can differentiate into embryonic and extra-embryonic cell types and are produced from the fusion of an egg and a sperm cell. Examples of these cells are the fertilized egg (zygote) and the cells at the immediate stages after fertilization. These cells develop into the cells that make up all the cells in an embryo and fetus. Totipotent cells are present only for a limited time as the fertilized egg and the cells produced by the first few divisions of the fertilized egg are totipotent. Totipotent stem cells give rise to somatic stem/progenitor cells and primitive germ-line stem cells.

Pluripotent Stem Cells: The true stem cell, these cells are considered the descendants of totipotent cells and can differentiate into nearly all cells. They are a blank canvas, possessing the ability for self-renewal and for differentiation into all cell types of the adult organism. Embryonic stem cells are the prime example of cells in this category.

Multipotent Stem Cells: While these stem cells are also considered true stem cells, they can only differentiate into a limited number of different cells that make up a closely related family of cells. In other words, they can give rise to other types of cells, but they have to keep it in the family: a particular tissue, organ, or physiological system. Examples of multipotent cells include:

- Bone marrow multipotent stem cells, which can give rise to all the cells of the blood but not to other types of cells.
- Stem cells found in adipose tissue.
- Stem cells that form multiple blood cell lineages.
- Adult stem cells and cord blood stem cells.

Oligopotent Stem Cells: These cells can differentiate into only a few cells. Examples include:

- Lymphoid (lymph) stem cells.
- Myeloid (bone marrow) stem cells.
- Corneal epithelium (the clear front surface of the eye) stem cells.

Unipotent Stem Cells: These can only produce their own cell type and possess the ability of self-renewal. This ability is what sets them apart from non-stem cells. Examples include:

- Muscle stem cells.

- Sperm-producing cells.

- Epithelial tissues, which self-renew with the help of unipotent progenitor cells.

Fetal Stem Cells: After ten weeks of gestation, the developing embryo is considered a fetus. These cells are currently categorized as adult stem cells; fetal stem cells are found in the organs, tissues, blood, and bone marrow of the fetus. Similar to adult stem cells, fetal stem cells are usually tissue-specific, and generate the mature cell types of the area where they reside. Although they are classified as adult stem cells, fetal tissues are different from other adult stem cells in that they contain pluripotent stem cells that promote the rapid growth and development of the organs. Another key difference is that fetal blood is rich in hematopoietic stem cells, which multiply at a pace more rapid than their counterparts found in cord blood or adult bone marrow.

Cord Blood Stem Cells: Umbilical cord blood contains some stem cells that are genetically identical to the infant. These cells are multipotent and can differentiate into certain, but not all, cell types. These cells are tissue-specific and can be used to create blood cells and cells of the immune system. Uses for cord blood stem cells include:

- Treat blood disorders, such as sickle cell anemia.

- Treat immune system conditions, such as leukemia.

- Restore the blood system after certain cancer treatments.

- Bank them for future stem cell therapy without fear of rejection.

- Donate them to those in need of an umbilical cord blood transplant to treat a variety of diseases.

Given the wide variety of regenerative abilities that the raw material of stem cells can offer, one can see the vast potential for new therapies to be developed for diseases such as diabetes and heart disease. Stem cell research can also shed light on new drug therapies or help us to understand the cause of birth defects. There is still much to learn, understand, and overcome with stem cells and over the past two decades we've seen new fields emerge, such as cell-based therapies and regenerative or reparative medicine.

Stem cell–based therapy may hold promise for previously untreatable diseases. Stem cell transplantation continues to be explored and researched as a potential therapy for debilitating neurodegenerative diseases, as a means to provide cell replacement or gene therapy. Diseases that may benefit from stem cell therapy include Alzheimer's disease, Parkinson's disease, Huntington's chorea, HIV-associated dementia, multiple sclerosis, amyotrophic lateral sclerosis, and even glaucoma. It is not far-fetched to imagine near-future treatments for broken bones or even osteoporosis by regenerating bone using cells originating from bone marrow stem cells, reversing type 1 diabetes by developing new insulin-producing pancreatic cells, repairing damaged nerves after a trauma, or using heart muscle stem cells to rebuild cardiac muscle after a heart attack.

Each new discovery can spur a new set of questions. However, unlike embryonic stem cells, adult stem cells seem to lose their ability to divide when removed from the body, making it a challenge to grow large amounts of adult stem cells in a laboratory setting. There is no doubt about the ethical questions that this field has generated; another whole book could be devoted entirely to this topic. For the purposes of this book on stem cell activation, however, we'll just touch on some of the main issues surrounding these miracle workers.

Ethical Considerations

The topic of stem cells can spur spirited ethical, political, moral, and religious debate, with certain types of stem cells taking more of the brunt of it than others. Adult stem cells and cord blood stem cells are now commonplace for use in research and clinical care. Some of the most common ethical issues regarding human embryonic stem cell research are concerns over the destruction of a human embryo, informed or voluntary consents, and the creation of an embryo for research purposes. Therapeutic cloning/SCNT also receives its share of objections. There is a high risk of genetic abnormalities, and the potential exists for severe congenital defects. Cloning humans, even if the science somehow made it possible to be done safely, also triggers questions about violating human dignity and the traditional, fundamental moral, religious, and cultural values that mankind possesses. Thoughts of human cloning becoming reality evoke images of Blade Runner and the "replicants." Maybe we can take a page from fiction and recognize that often when we mess with Mother Nature things usually do not go well. The cloning of human embryos for reproductive purposes is largely viewed as morally reprehensible and is illegal in a number of states. Some people feel this technique should be banned because the technology exists for SCNT to be used for human reproduction.

Advances in the research—with induced pluripotent stem cells (iPSCs) and their limitless differentiation potential—raises ethical questions regarding human cloning. Furthermore, while mesenchymal stem cells (see page 19) have numerous clinical uses and positive benefits, especially with autoimmune and chronic inflammatory diseases, there is still much to be learned as these cells have been shown to possess the capability to encourage tumor growth and metastasis. These concerns contribute to some of the ethical and safety challenges faced by researchers and providers in the growing field of regenerative medicine.

You may have your own strong feelings about these issues, and there are no easy answers to the ethical questions that are raised. Where should the line in the sand be drawn? At what point do we upset the balance of survival of the fittest and Darwinian theories of evolution? We are not here for philosophical debates, however, so let's get back to learning about the purposes for and applications of stem cells.

What Are Stem Cells Used For?

Stem cell therapy holds great potential for the repair of damaged or injured tissues and organs. In order to appreciate our forthcoming discussion on how diet and lifestyle changes can optimize your stem cells, we need to continue exploring the science and biology behind these miracle workers.

Remember we discussed the three qualities that make these cells unique.

1. They are unspecialized. Stem cells lack any tissue-specific structures that would give the ability to perform a specific task or function. A stem cell will not stand alongside a nerve cell and work to transmit a nerve signal.

2. They can divide and renew themselves for long periods of time. Embryonic stem cells can proliferate for over a year in lab settings and a small population of cells can grow into millions.

3. They can develop into specialized cell types.

- While a stem cell won't work alongside another type of cell, it *can* become one of those other specialized cells through the process of cell differentiation.

- Cell differentiation is a step-by-step process controlled by signals occurring within and outside of the cell.

- Internally the signals are controlled by genes and the coded map of instructions carried on DNA. This roadmap details cell structure and function.

- Externally, the signals are provided by chemicals given off by other cells, molecules in the stem cell's fluid environment, and the other cells with which the stem cell may be in physical contact.

- This dance of signals during the process of differentiation can impact what regulating proteins in the cell's DNA get turned on or off and can affect DNA expression, which is called an epigenetic mark.

Within the categories of stem cells, embryonic and adult, there are numerous different types of cells. For the purpose of this book, we'll focus our attention on optimizing adult stem cells.

Adult stem cells *usually* create the cell types of the tissue in which they dwell. For example, adult stem cells include blood stem cells, which reside in the bone marrow and produce red blood cells and white blood cells, whereas neural stem cells will create new neurons. Research on adult stem cells has shown that these cells exist in many organ systems and tissues throughout the body. Stem cells are thought to "hang out" in tissues in an area called a "stem cell niche."

There is also current evidence showing that some stem cells are *pericytes*, which are cells involved in maintaining the structural integrity of the layers of blood vessels. We know that stem cells possess the ability to be quiescent (or hang out) for extended periods until they are called upon and activated to generate or regenerate cells because of normal wear and tear, or in response to disease or tissue injury.

As stem cells have been found in the skin, teeth, brain, bone marrow, bloodstream, blood vessels, skeletal muscle, heart, gut, liver, and reproductive tissues such as the ovarian epithelium (female nipple) and testis (male reproductive gland), just imagine the possibilities for health and longevity if we learn how best to optimize the activation of these cells.

Adult Stem Cell Types and Function

Hematopoietic stem cells (HSCs): Create all the types of red, white, and lymphocytic blood cells.

- white blood cells include natural killer cells, which help fight cancer and viruses; neutrophils, which fight infections and injury; basophils, which help the immune system function; eosinophils, which fight disease; monocytes, which can differentiate into different types of white blood cells; and macrophages, which can travel to infection sights.

- lymphocytic cells include B lymphocytes and T lymphocytes, which activate the immune system to destroy pathogens.

Mesenchymal stem cells (MSCs): Are present in many tissues.

- A very rich source of these cells is the developing tooth bud of the mandibular third molar.

- Those in the bone marrow, bone marrow stromal stem cells, and skeletal stem cells will create a variety of cell types.

  - bone cells—osteoblasts and osteocytes

  - cartilage cells—chondrocytes

  - fat cells—adipocytes

  - stromal cells that help the formation of blood

Neural stem cells: Create the three major cell types found in the brain.

- Nerve cells—neurons

- Two categories of non-neuronal cells—astrocytes and oligodendrocytes

Epithelial stem cells: Found deep in the lining of the digestive tract and create several cell types.

- absorptive cells—also known as enterocytes, they are the most common epithelial cell type lining the lumen, which is the lining of the small intestine and colon. These cells are highly specialized with the job of absorption and transportation of nutrients across plasma membranes.

- goblet cells—cells that produce mucus in the lining of the GI tract

- Paneth cells—located in your intestinal crypts (think of these as "the pockets in your intestines"), these cells secrete anti-bacterial proteins which protect the stem cells that line the walls of the crypt.

- enteroendocrine cells—a class of epithelial cells mixed in with the absorptive and exocrine cells that line the digestive tract. They are usually found in the gastric glands and intestinal crypts. These cells secrete specific hormones that impact intestinal secretions and motility.

Skin stem cells: Present in the basal layer of the epidermis and at the base of hair follicles.

- Epidermal stem cells create keratinocytes, the cells that produce the protein keratin, which helps to give our skin its flexibility and strength.

- Follicular stem cells create both the hair follicle and the epidermis.

Earlier, I mentioned that adult stem cells *usually* create cells within the types of tissue where they reside. One area of stem cell research that warrants much more attention based on the limited current body of evidence is the phenomenon known as *transdifferentiation*.

Transdifferentiation is when an adult stem cell differentiates into a type of cell other than what is anticipated based on the tissue of origin. For example, if a blood stem cell gives rise to a cardiac muscle cell, or a brain stem cell gives rise to a red blood cell.

Another exciting area for further research into adult stem cells is the process of *reprogramming*. Reprogramming is when, through a genetic modification process, an adult stem cell can be turned into other types of cells. Through this process exists the opportunity to use existing cells to create cells of another type that may have become damaged or lost. Reprogramming can also result in the creation of iPSCs (see page 11 for definition).

While iPSCs will continue to be the subject of more research, they have already shown promise and utility in the development of new pharmacological agents and in expanding our understanding of the pathophysiology of certain diseases. There is still a long road yet to travel before iPSCs become commonplace therapies.

Much of the buzz around the future of iPSCs is how to "de-differentiate" cells. Studies on reprogramming include viral and non-viral methods. Unfortunately, in some animal models, viral reprogramming led to the development of cancers. One positive note for the future of tissues derived from iPSCs is they will come with a reduced risk of rejection as they will practically be an identical match to the cell donor. The hopeful future of iPSC research is that we can one day possess the knowledge and capability to reprogram cells in order to repair damaged tissues in our body.

Stem Cell Transplants

Although there is currently a heightened focus on stem cells, some of these treatments have been around for decades, and with a good track record. For example, adult stem cell therapies developed from bone marrow transplants have been used to treat blood and bone cancers such as leukemia. Veterinary medicine has also benefited from advances in stem cell applications. Adult stem cells are used in horses as a treatment for tendon and ligament injuries. We previously discussed how our adult stem cells undergo rapid production when called upon to regenerate the specialized tissues. Isolating and using one's own adult stem cells could help to reduce many of the immunological side effects and rejection issues seen with cell transplant.

This, in turn, reduces the need for immunosuppressive drugs, which in many cases cause their own side effects.

No crash course on stem cells would be complete without giving you an overview on the two basic types of stem cell transplants. They are autologous and allogeneic.

Autologous Stem Cell Transplant

There are two types of autologous stem cell transplant: autologous hematopoietic stem cell transplantation, and mesenchymal stem cell transplantation. They are generally associated with cancer treatment for leukemia, lymphoma, pediatric cancer, and multiple myeloma. With this type of transplant the patient self-donates his or her own stem cells before beginning cancer treatment. The stem cells are obtained from either bone marrow or blood and then frozen. After chemo or radiation therapy, the stem cells are given back to the patient. As discussed previously, the advantage of self-donation/autologous stem cell transplant is that when you receive your own cells, there is no risk of transplant rejection. Autologous platelet-rich plasma (PRP) falls into this category and is used in the treatment of tissue defects.

Key Points on Hematopoietic Stem Cell Transplantation

- HSCs are the most commonly transplanted adult stem cells.

- They're used for the treatment of numerous genetic and acquired diseases such as blood cancers, autoimmune disorders, and hematopoietic defects.

- In treating severe autoimmune diseases, favorable results have been achieved using high-dose immunosuppressive therapy with autologous hematopoietic stem cell transplantation.

- Because this type of cell possesses the ability to regenerate, HSCs are well suited for gene therapies.

Key Points on Mesenchymal Stem Cell Transplantation

- MSCs are used for cell therapy in the treatment of numerous neurological disorders.

- Qualities of MSCs include:

  - The cells are self-renewable.

  - They can be obtained from embryonic or bone marrow and adipose tissue.

  - Bone marrow-derived mesenchymal stem cells can differentiate into several cell types.

  - Adult MSCs are useful as a therapy for cartilage regeneration.

Allogeneic Stem Cell Transplant

A key difference in the allogeneic stem cell transplant is that the stem cells come from a donor, not the patient. Allogeneic transplants are used for a variety of diseases but are most commonly used to treat certain types of leukemia, lymphoma, and other bone marrow disorders such as myelodysplasia. A histocompatible (tissue compatible) donor is required, so the donor is preferably a family member or someone whose tissue type is a close match to the recipient.

Allogeneic stem cell transplantation has a different set of advantages from an autologous stem cell transplant. One such advantage is, once a match is found, a donor can be asked to donate white blood cells and more stem cells as necessary. These cells from a healthy donor are also cancer-free cells. Another key advantage is that donor stem cells make their own immune cells, and after a high-dose treatment, this immune response creates a situation called the graft-versus-cancer effect. The benefit here is that it can assist in destroying any remaining cancer cells. Umbilical cord and placental blood have become newer sources of stem cells in this category.

A Note on Syngeneic Stem Cell Transplant

- The syngeneic stem cell transplant is a special type of allogeneic transplant that only occurs when the donor and recipient are identical twins or identical triplets.

- Graft-versus-host disease is not an issue. GVHD is caused by an immune condition after a transplant procedure when immune cells from the donor (the graft or graft cells) attack the recipient's (patient) own tissues (as they are the host). While considered to be a rare side effect that can occur at any time post-transplant, it is most commonly seen in allogeneic bone marrow/stem cell transplant.

Stem Cell Media Buzz

With the increase in knowledge and application of stem cell therapies, combined with the slow decline in costs associated with some of these treatments, we're seeing more and more regenerative medicine centers and an entire industry focused on delivering therapies like platelet-rich plasma (see page 27) and various stem cell treatments. How often are you bombarded with ads or commercials about the next information session to be held at Hotel A to discuss Dr. B's clinic using product C to heal you of X, Y, and Z? Many of these programs are aimed at providing what is now commonly referred to as regenerative medicine.

Regenerative Medicine Defined

The NIH defines regenerative medicine as "the process of creating living, functional tissues to repair or replace tissue or organ function lost due to age, disease, damage, or congenital defects."[3] This fast-growing specialty in medicine includes the creation of stem cells for therapeutic use, as well as the engineering of tissues and the production of artificial organs.

In regenerative medicine research, scientists are conducting experiments in laboratory settings where they can literally create, grow, and develop tissues and organs with the goal of safely transplanting them when the body has lost the ability to heal on its own. Bladders that have been grown from the patient's own cells can be successfully transplanted. Imagine the possibilities here!

As of January 2019, statistics on organ donation show there were more than 113,000 people on the national transplant waiting list. It is estimated that twenty people die each day while waiting on a transplant list. Regenerative medicine can chart a course to where those lists no longer exist. I find myself thinking back to the sci-fi movies I watched as a kid, like *The Thing* and *Invasion of the Body Snatchers:* Cutting-edge science is making science-fact out of what previously was just imagination and science-fiction. It may sound creepy and weird, but this field has been around for decades. During my days in the home infusion industry, I had the opportunity to deal with teams who performed multivisceral transplants, surgeries where multiple organs are transplanted at once, usually including the liver, small intestine, pancreas, and sometimes the stomach and part of the large intestine.

I too am a recipient of the advances regenerative medicine has provided. In 2013 when the large tumor was removed from my

---

3   National Institute of Health Fact Sheets, "Regenerative Medicine."

left abdominal wall, I lost my entire left rectus muscle and part of my left obliques. As part of the comprehensive rebuilding of my abdomen, my brilliant surgeons used a biological mesh made with tissue from pigs along with muscle tissue from my right side to help reinforce the area on my left side that was now missing some major structural support.

Transplant surgeries have come a long way since the first procedures done in the early twentieth century when success was seen with bone, cornea, and soft tissue transplants. In the mid-1950's we saw the first successful solid organ transplants using kidneys, and the following decades saw continuing advances in organ and tissue transplants, and even living donor transplantation. Today it's commonplace for wounds, burns, and issues like diabetic ulcers to be treated with tissue-engineered skin. We also see these products being used in orthopedic procedures and even in heart surgeries.

So, where do stem cells fit into all this? Remember that these miracle worker cells are programmed to generate, regenerate, and renew our bodies so they hold infinite possibilities and currently are used to increase the type and use of engineered tissues. Therefore, we're not too far off from the sci-fi images of growing new body parts to replace old, worn-out, or damaged ones. In fact, tissue-engineering research combined with advancements in 3-D printing has led to a new technique called "organ printing."

By now, you may be thinking about your medical history and possibly even parts of your body that may be in need of repair or replacement. Have those regenerative medicine ads and commercials caught your eye? Many of those clinics advertising that they can repair and restore your body, reduce your pain, regrow your hair, and rejuvenate your skin are using platelet-rich plasma and stem cell–based therapies. One important note here is many health insurance plans consider these treatments experimental or investigational and, therefore, may not cover them. Before signing on for any of these treatments, be sure to inquire about what your individual plan's benefits are.

Platelet-Rich Plasma (PRP)

PRP is made through a process using your own blood. Whole blood is made up of red blood cells, white blood cells, platelets, and plasma. Platelets are needed to form blood clots, and they contain growth factors that are vital to your body's normal healing process. In fact, the ability of a wound to heal its damaged tissues depends on the platelet concentrations. Platelets are the first cell type to arrive on the scene of tissue injury and are especially active in the beginning stages of inflammation and the healing process.

Plasma is the liquid portion of whole blood, made up mostly of water and proteins. When someone is preparing for PRP injections, a few vials of their own blood with be drawn and then spun down in a centrifuge, which helps to separate the cells from the plasma. Platelets are then concentrated to two to five times the normal amount found in whole blood and injected into the injured or diseased area. The goal of the injection for tissue repair is to optimize the healing powers of the growth factors in the platelets and fibrinogen (a clotting factor protein vital for blood clots to properly form) in the plasma.

PRP is currently being used as a therapeutic option for wound healing and numerous conditions such as tendon, ligament, muscle, and cartilage injuries; early osteoarthritis; improving an existing scar's appearance; rejuvenating skin for a more youthful appearance; and treating alopecia, or hair loss. Current research has helped to improve our understanding of the job description of platelets. Where it was previously thought that their primary duty was blood clot formation, research has confirmed that platelets can assist with controlling inflammation and forming new blood vessels (angiogenesis), as well as the movement of stem cells within the body and rapid increases in cell numbers. It is important to note that not all PRP is the same, and currently there exists a lack of a standardized protocol for preparation.

Other areas where PRP is currently being used and/or researched include maxillofacial (facial or jaw) and oral surgery, cleft lip and palate in children, cardiac surgery, plastic surgery, ophthalmology, and dermatology, as well as urological and gynecological applications. An advantage of using PRP is how quickly the injection can be prepared immediately after having your own blood drawn. It does not need to be preserved in any facility, which helps to reduce the associated costs involved with this treatment. Additionally, since it is made utilizing your own cells, it will not trigger an immune response and the risk of exposure to bloodborne contaminations is reduced.

There are not many disadvantages associated with the use of PRP, but as with any therapy and injection, there always exists some degree of risk. These risks include injection-site morbidity. infection or injury to nerves or blood vessels near the injection site, and possibly, a blood clot.

Instances of the development of a scar or calcification at the site of the injection have also been reported. There are certain individuals for which PRP may not be the best option. For example, anyone with a weakened immune system or with certain predisposed diseases will have a higher risk of developing an infection at the injury site. Certain lifestyle choices, such as chronic smoking, or drug or alcohol use, may also cause a provider to advise against using PRP. Those with a medical history of blood disorders, liver disease, frequent infections, use of blood thinner medications, cancer, metabolic disorders, chronic skin conditions, or systemic disorders may not be good candidates for PRP due to increased risk for complications.

Despite a body of clinical studies illustrating the benefits of PRP, they have not yet received approval from the Food and Drug Administration. Presently, PRP is considered safe as well as natural, but the commonly reported side effect is temporary pain and swelling in the treatment area. In general, adverse reactions are very low, and more research is needed to determine the long-term effectiveness of PRP as well as its possible long-term side effects.

Stem Cell Therapy

Stem cell therapy has shown promise where traditional medicines may have failed. The therapy's unique qualities show great promise to replace cells that are no longer working or are damaged or diseased. Unlike PRP, stem cells are identified in adult tissues then isolated and cultured in a clinical setting, where it takes weeks for them to grow before they can be used in a therapeutic manner. Although PRP can be used much more quickly than stem cell therapy, the curative ability of PRP is markedly lower than that of stem cell therapy.

The differences between platelet-rich plasma and stem-cell therapy are summarized in the following table:

CHARACTERISTIC FEATURES	PRP	STEM CELL THERAPY
What is the source of the cells and their makeup?	Venous blood. Made up of various growth factors and cytokines.	Bone marrow, embryo, other body tissues. Made of undifferentiated cells.
How does the treatment work?	Action of anti-inflammatory and regenerative potential.	Cells differentiate into many cell types determined by the site. Anti-inflammatory, immunosuppressive, regenerates tissues and bone.
How effective is the treatment?	Greater efficacy in younger patients, minimal side effects.	Greater efficacy than with PRP. A common therapy for osteoarthritis.
What are the potential complications?	Less reported minor adverse effects compared to stem cell therapy. No major side effects.	Pain and swelling is most common. In theory, it may increase one's risk of cancer, but evidence to support this is lacking.

Stem cells are harvested either from fat tissue or bone marrow. In some cases, stem cells are used together with your platelets. Even after being isolated, these cells still hold onto their power to become any number of a variety of different cells found in the body.

We discussed how stem cells possess the ability to self-renew and the power to differentiate into about 200 different cell types found in the adult body. Additionally, stem cells produce certain growth factors and cytokines (small proteins that are secreted, which have a specific effect on how cells interact and communicate with one another) that speed up the healing process at the site of tissue injury or damage. While PRP aims to harness the healing properties within platelets, stem cell therapies in regenerative medicine focus on replacing damaged cells and can be used in conditions where PRP would not yield any benefits.

We still have a lot left to learn and research about the power behind stem cell therapy, but one thing we know for sure is just how powerful stem cells can be in our immune system and in the regulation of this system. Advantages of stem cell therapy include the ability of the cells to be directly obtained from the intended recipient (autologous transplantation), the fact that the number of cells obtained from a single retrieval can yield a lifetime's worth of cells for that individual, and the ability of stem cells to be manipulated through genetic modification to force the expression of certain genes that would help facilitate improved wound healing and decrease the likelihood of scarring.

The study of stem cells has shown us exactly how strongly influenced the cells are by their surroundings, thereby impacting their ability to self renew or to differentiate into other cells. One disadvantage of stem therapy is, this influence can make it difficult for clinicians to determine the difference between how a particular culture of cells will behave *in vitro* versus *in vivo*. The stem cells should always be differentiated into the intended cell types before they are used therapeutically. Another disadvantage: the survival rates of stem cells retrieved and isolated can be low, especially given variables such as laboratory personnel skill levels and adherence to procedures that reduce the risk of contamination.

Even though stem cell therapy holds a cornucopia of promise, we cannot ignore some of the potential risks. For example, there is evidence showing that MSCs obtained from fat cells lose genetic stability over time and are likely to develop tumors.

Without knowing all of the long-term risks, it goes without saying that patients who have undergone stem cell therapy will require long-term follow-up.

Things to Consider about Stem Cell Therapies

Marketing and advertising may seem as if they are outpacing the current level of knowledge and research for stem cell injectables. So, a word of caution: If something sounds too good to be true, it probably is. There are many unproven treatments being marketed in the US and around the world, and they can be dangerous to your health. Get all of the available facts before receiving any treatments.

The FDA's advice for anyone considering stem cell therapies is as follows:

1. Know that the FDA plays a role in stem cell treatment oversight. You may be told that because these are your cells, the FDA does not need to review or approve the treatment. That is not true.

2. Stem cell products have the potential to treat many medical conditions and diseases. But for almost all of these products, it is not yet known whether the product has any benefit—or if the product is safe to use. If you're considering treatment in the United States:

- Ask if the FDA has reviewed the treatment. Ask your health care provider to confirm this information. You also can ask the clinical investigator to give you the FDA-issued Investigational New Drug Application number and the chance to review the FDA communication acknowledging the IND. Ask for this information *before* getting treatment— even if the stem cells are your own.

- Request the facts and ask questions if you don't understand. To participate in a clinical trial that requires an IND application, you must sign a consent form that explains the experimental procedure. The consent form also identifies the Institutional Review Board that assures the protection of the rights and welfare of human subjects. Make sure you understand the entire process and known risks before you sign. You also can ask the study sponsor for the clinical investigator's brochure, which includes a short description of the product and information about its safety and effectiveness.

If you're considering treatment in another country:

- Learn about regulations that cover products in that country.

- Know that the FDA does not have oversight of treatments done in other countries. The FDA typically has little information about foreign establishments or their stem cell products.

- Be cautious. If you're considering a stem cell–based product in a country that may not require regulatory review of clinical studies, it may be hard to know if the experimental treatment is reasonably safe.

In this chapter, we've covered exactly how important stem cells are because of their job: to *generate, regenerate, and renew* your body. We also discussed the future of stem cell research, working toward the goal that we can one day possess the knowledge and capability to reprogram cells in order to repair damaged tissues in the body. What if instead of waiting for that research to be completed, you started making changes today that could tap into your current stem cells' ability to *generate, regenerate, and renew* your body and take back control over your health?

Chapter 2

THE STATE OF THE AMERICAN DIET

Before we can delve into the ways we can use diet to tap into the restorative possibilities of our stem cells, we should cover a few nutrition basics. Also this will set the groundwork for our later discussions.

Nutrition Basics

Nutrients are divided into two categories: macronutrients and micronutrients. Macronutrients are those nutrients that the body needs in large quantities. They are carbohydrates, proteins, and fats. Macronutrients also provide the body with fuel in the form of caloric energy. The analogy that I use to describe macronutrients to a client is that we are essentially trying to build and maintain a structure—our bodies. Carbohydrates and fats are the construction workers, and protein is the main construction material. Carbohydrates and fats provide fuel in the form of caloric energy so that they can make use of your construction material, proteins. Proteins provide the building material in the form of amino acids, referred to as the "building blocks" for protein.

In recent years we have seen a heightened awareness of manipulating one's "macros" to conform to whichever trendy diet someone may be trying to follow. While we are not going to get into a debate here over each style of diet that is popular in our culture, I do want to stress that when you are trying to be efficient and building a structure, you generally do not want to end up burning your building material (proteins) as a fuel source. Therefore, one of my biggest pet peeves about many popular diet plans is the high amounts of proteins they encourage while restricting adequate amounts of carbohydrates and/or fats. In order to spare your protein construction materials, you will need adequate construction workers in the form of carbohydrates or fats. This is where personalized nutrition recommendations become pivotal because there is no one-size-fits-all approach to nutrition and diet. In my opinion, there isn't even a one-size-fits-most approach.

Some people thrive on a higher-carbohydrate, lower-fat diet. However, others are quite the opposite and can do much better on a higher-fat, lower-carbohydrate plan. Consider your body's metabolism in terms of a campfire. We usually start off with tinder and kindling to get a fire going, but it's the larger logs that will burn the longest. Each fire may need a different amount of tinder, kindling, and larger logs to burn long, efficiently, and produce heat. Simple carbohydrates are your tinder, complex carbohydrates are the kindling, and healthy fats are your logs. You may be asking, where does protein fit here? Ideally, your protein intake is not meant to be used for fuel, therefore we don't want to burn our protein calories for energy.

Each of us needs to find the right combination of the three to keep our individual fires burning brightly. Another caveat to personalization would be to consider any food allergies, sensitivities, or intolerances (but that's a topic for an entirely separate book).

Bear in mind though, increasing your consumption of one macronutrient often results in decreases of another, and the potential then exists for insufficiencies to occur. Therefore, two things that must be emphasized regardless of which style of diet you subscribe to are: (1) quality counts—quality always trumps quantity and (2) variety is the spice of life. The best way to ensure nutrient density is to eat a variety of foods. The theme here is EAT REAL FOOD! Consider this, are there certain foods that you would not feel comfortable feeding to a child, maybe because you would classify them as "unhealthy" or a "poor choice"? If so, do you consume those foods yourself? If you answered "yes," why would you want to eat something that you felt was not healthy?

Snapshot of Macronutrients

Carbohydrates

- Provide four calories per gram
- Considered to be the body's preferred fuel source
- Can be stored in the body for later use as energy
- The liver and muscles store carbohydrate in the form of glycogen (although our body's main form of stored fuel is fat).
- Carbohydrates exist in three main forms: sugar, starch, and fiber.
- A good rule of thumb: If it comes from a plant, it's a source of carbohydrates. Therefore, they are found in fruits, grains, vegetables, beans, legumes, and even nuts and seeds.

- Some dairy products such as milk, kefir, and yogurts contain carbohydrates.

- Spare protein to preserve the body's lean muscle mass

Tips for choosing carbohydrate-containing foods (you may need to alter these based on your own personal tolerances):

1. Know the difference between simple and complex carbohydrates. They differ by chemistry and rate of digestion and absorption.

Simple carbohydrates/sugars have one or two sugars. They will be broken down and absorbed quickly. These can cause rapid rises in blood sugar (blood glucose), even if you're not a diabetic. Candy, sweeteners, soda, and syrups fall into this category. (Ever heard a food referred to as "empty calories"? They bring the calories but not much else of worth to the party.) Limit your consumption of simple sugars:

- Monosaccharides (one sugar molecule): fructose and galactose

- Disaccharides (two sugar molecules): sucrose, lactose, and maltose

Complex carbohydrates have three or more sugar molecules and are referred to as polysaccharides or starches. These carbs will take longer to be digested and absorbed, therefore getting you fuller longer while also helping to keep blood glucose levels more stable.

- Vegetables, beans, peas, lentils, and whole grains are complex carbohydrates.

2. Aim for unprocessed or minimally processed.

- Avoid the white stuff: sugar, white breads, and white flours. Consider these to be naked grains. The other coverings have been removed in processing, along with fiber and some key nutritional value. Even monitor how often you eat white starches like potatoes and white rice.

- Look for whole grain, which is a step above whole wheat.

- Get familiar with food labels, ingredient lists, and nutrition facts. If you see less than 3 grams of fiber in a grain-based cereal, bread, or cracker, choose one with more fiber.

- If you see the term "enriched" then you know the manufacturer tried to replace nutrients that were lost in processing—reg flag!

- Consume at least 25 grams of fiber per day.

- Better yet, go for the items that don't come in packaging or need a nutrition facts label. Stick to the outer perimeter produce section of your grocery store.

- Aim for items that naturally come from plants, not those made in manufacturing plants!

- Remember, quality counts! I encourage my clients to opt for organic and non-GMO foods as much as realistically possible for them. No fake foods!

Proteins

- Provide four calories per gram

- Are the workhorse of the cell

- Needed for structure, regulation, and function of the body's cells, tissues, and organs, as well as metabolic, transport, and hormone systems

- Components of cell plasma membranes

Tips for choosing protein-containing foods (you may need to alter these based on your own personal tolerances):

1. Remember quality still counts here too!

2. Consider eating more organic, non-GMO, plant-based protein sources: legumes like beans and peas, lentils, spirulina, nutritional yeast, and nuts and seeds. How about opting for meatless Mondays to get you started with more plant-based foods?

3. If/when you are choosing animal protein, aim for lean, organic, free-range, grass-fed, wild-caught, or low mercury as often as you can.

4. Eggs, cheese, poultry, seafood/fish, yes—even beef and pork are good sources of protein, just be sure to choose quality sources.

5. Dairy products like milk, kefir, and yogurt pull double duty providing protein and carbohydrates.

6. I repeat, no fake foods! (That includes all the recent hype over fast food burgers that are "plant based.")

Fats

- Provide nine calories per gram
- An essential fuel source
- Support cell growth
- Protect organs
- Aid in body temperature regulation and providing insulation
- Provide transportation and absorption of certain nutrients

- Necessary for the synthesis of hormones and neurotransmitters

Tips for choosing fat-containing foods (you may need to alter these based on your own personal tolerances):

1. Quality continues to matter here too, so look for minimally refined, organic, cold-pressed, non-GMO as often as you can.

2. Lose the fat-shaming mentality of the latter portion of the twentieth century, and don't blame the butter for what the white bread and hash browns did!

3. Let me say it again: No fake foods, especially fake fats. Let's leave the processed oils, fat substitutes, margarines, spreads, and shortening in the last century where it belongs and will never rot (insert time capsule mental images here).

4. Wild-caught, low mercury, cold-water fish are an excellent source of your healthy omega-3 fatty acids. The fish most associated with high levels of mercury include shark, bigeye tuna, swordfish, king mackerel, tile fish, bass, walleye, and pickerel.

5. Opt for whole food natural fats like olives, avocados, coconut, real butter, quality dairy fat (no skim/fat free or 1%/low-fat dairy is allowed in my house), and nuts or seeds.

6. Let's just clear the air on animal fats, especially beef—quality does make a difference. The fatty acid profile of conventional beef has a much higher content of omega-6 fatty acids (which are considered to be pro-inflammatory and consumed in excess in the American diet) than grass-fed beef.

7. Be judicious with your choice of oils. Always give your oils (even nuts and seeds) a sniff test. When in doubt of rancidity, throw it out. Also, try to avoid the big-box store jumbo bottle;

it'll most likely go rancid before you get to use it all. For cooking oils, I use heavier oils such as avocado oil, butter, ghee, virgin coconut oil, and extra-virgin olive oil (EVOO). These are more stable fats and can hold up to higher heat, with the exception of EVOO, which is best for medium, not high heat.

8. Lighter and more delicate oils, such as nut or seed oils—almond, flaxseed, grapeseed, hempseed, sesame, sunflower, walnut, etc.—are best for lower temperature cooking/baking, salad dressings, or where a lighter flavor is desired. If you choose to use safflower or sunflower oils be sure to use those labeled high-oleic.

Snapshot of Micronutrients

Micronutrients are those nutrients that the body needs in smaller amounts. These include water-soluble and fat-soluble vitamins. Water-soluble vitamins include ascorbic acid (vitamin C) and the B vitamins—thiamin, riboflavin, niacin, vitamin B6 (pyridoxine, pyridoxal, and pyridoxamine), folacin, vitamin B12, biotin, and pantothenic acid.

Fat-soluble vitamins include vitamins A, D, E, and K, macrominerals, trace minerals, and water. Are you ready to revisit high school chemistry and biology classes?

Water-Soluble Vitamins: Job Duties and Food Sources

Water-soluble vitamins, as their name suggests, dissolve in water. These essential vitamins are carried to your body's tissues. However the body stores little to none of these vitamins in the body. In order for your body to use these vitamins, they must be absorbed. Factors that can influence absorption include the vitamin source (natural or synthetic), food source quality and composition, preparation method, how well digestion is working, and baseline nutritional status. Changes related to any of these factors can lead to decreased absorption. Therefore, any excess or nonabsorbed vitamins will pass through and be excreted. (Yes, I mean that you'll pee or poop out the extras, so if you're someone who has been over-supplementing, there's a good chance you're contributing to the vitamin density of your local sewer or septic system.)

As for food preparation, numerous methods can be used. For example, foods may be boiled, parboiled, blanched, steamed, pureed, baked, roasted, sautéed, fried, broiled, and/or micro-waved. I sincerely hope you are not relying heavily on the microwave as clinical research has shown how microwaving foods decreases their nutrient composition. Remember, vitamins are heat sensitive, so the amount, type, and length of heat exposure will affect the nutrient's bioavailability. Also, nutrients will leach out in fluids, either those they are stored in (canned vegetables, for example) or water vegetables are boiled in. When you toss the liquids, lost vitamins will be contained in the fluid.

Vitamin B1 (thiamine): Part of the coenzyme thiamin pyrophosphate (coenzymes or cofactors are compounds that are necessary for an enzyme to do its job). Assists in energy metabolism and carbohydrate conversion. Involved in nerve and muscle activity. Also considered to be a nutrient linked with digestion, skin, hair, eyes, mouth, liver, and the immune system.

Sources: pork, organ meats, beans, peas, whole grains, brown rice, wheat germ, bran, Brewer's yeast, blackstrap molasses, nuts, and sunflower seeds

Vitamin B2 (riboflavin): Serves as a coenzyme in energy metabolism and carbohydrate conversion. It is involved in growth and development and red blood cell formation.

Sources: Brewer's yeast, almonds, meats, organ meats, whole grains, wheat germ, mushrooms, soy, dairy, eggs, spinach, and oysters

Vitamin B3 (niacin): Involved in cholesterol production, conversion of food into energy, digestion, and nervous system function. The body can manufacture niacin from tryptophan.

Sources: beans, beets, Brewer's yeast, meats, poultry, organ meats, fish, seeds, nuts, and whole grains

Vitamin B5 (pantothenic acid): Involved in the conversion of food into energy, fat metabolism, sex and stress-related hormone production, nervous system function, red blood cell formation, immune function, and healthy digestion. Helps the body to use other nutrients.

Sources: meats, vegetables, whole grains, legumes, lentils, egg yolks, milk, sweet potatoes, seeds, nuts, wheat germ, and salmon

Vitamin B6 (pyridoxine): Works with immune and nervous system function; protein, carbohydrate, and fat metabolism; and red blood cell production. Involved with DNA/RNA and B12 absorption. Reduces homocysteine; an elevated homocysteine level is a risk factor for cardiac disease and is often associated with low levels of B vitamins, particularly B6, B12, and folate. It can also be caused by kidney issues, psoriasis, decreased thyroid hormone, and certain medications.

Sources: poultry, tuna, salmon, shrimp, beef liver, lentils, soybeans, chickpeas, seeds, nuts, avocados, bananas, carrots, brown rice, bran, wheat germ, and whole grain flour

Vitamin B7 (biotin): Involved in energy storage, and protein, carbohydrate, and fat metabolism.

Sources: salmon, liver, pork, avocados, cauliflower, raspberries, whole grains, legumes, lentils, egg yolks, milk, sweet potatoes, seeds, nuts, and wheat germ

Vitamin B9 (folate/folic acid): Flagged as a nutrient of concern due to inadequate intake, especially for women of child-bearing age. Involved in mental health and prevention of birth defects in infant DNA/RNA. Works with B12 to regulate red blood cell production and iron function. Reduces homocysteine.

Sources: asparagus, avocado, fortified grains, tomato juice, green leafy vegetables, black-eyed peas, lentils, beans, and orange juice

Vitamin B12 (cobalamin): Works on conversion of food into energy, nervous system function, red blood cell formation, iron function, DNA/RNA synthesis. Can be a nutrient of concern in poorly planned vegan/vegetarian diet, those with low stomach acid, and those on long-term proton pump inhibitor (PPI) medication.

Sources: fish and seafood, meats, poultry, eggs, dairy products, and fortified cereals

Vitamin C (ascorbic acid): Functions as an antioxidant, involved in collagen and tissue formation, wound healing, immune function, enzyme activation, transmitting hormonal information, blood clotting, cell and cell organelle membrane function, nerve impulse transmission, and muscular contraction and tone. Prevents weakness and irritability.

Sources: broccoli, Brussels sprouts, cantaloupe, cauliflower, citrus, guava, kiwi, papaya, parsley, peas, potatoes, peppers, parsley, rose hips, strawberries, and tomatoes

Fat-Soluble Vitamins: Job Duties and Food Sources

Fat-soluble vitamins, as the name implies, are dissolved in fat before they are absorbed. Unlike with the water-soluble vitamins, extras or excesses of these vitamins are stored in the liver and fat tissue, and they are usually not destroyed by cooking methods.

Vitamin A: Necessary for vision, immune function, skin and bone formation, essential cell growth and development, reproduction, and red blood cell formation.

Sources: dairy, eggs, liver, fortified cereals, carrots, cantaloupe, green leafy vegetables, fruits, pumpkin, red peppers, and sweet potatoes

Vitamin D: Required to maintain normal blood levels of calcium and phosphate, which is necessary for normal bone mineralization, muscle contraction, nerve conduction, and general cellular function in all body cells. Vitamin D also impacts hormone and neurotransmitter production, immune function, and blood pressure regulation. Vitamin D is flagged as a nutrient of concern due to the prevalence of clinical deficiencies and insufficiencies and especially for those on long-term PPI medications.

Sources: sunlight, fortified dairy products, fish liver oil, fortified cereals, fortified orange juice, egg yolks, liver, fish, and fortified soy beverages

Vitamin E: Functions as an antioxidant, regulates oxidation reactions, stabilizes cell membrane, aids in the formation of blood vessels, helps with immune function, and protects against cardiovascular disease, cataracts, and macular degeneration.

Sources: wheat germ, liver, eggs, nuts, seeds, cold-pressed vegetable oils, dark leafy greens, sweet potatoes, avocados, asparagus, peanuts, peanut butter, and fortified cereals and juices

Vitamin K: Aids in blood clotting and bone proteins. Also works on the formation of glucose into glycogen for storage in the liver.

Sources: green vegetables like kale, turnip greens, spinach, broccoli, lettuce, and cabbage, beef liver, asparagus, watercress, cheese, oats, peas, whole wheat, and green tea

Macrominerals: Job Duties and Food Sources

Calcium: Involved in blood clotting, bone and teeth formation, blood vessel constriction and relaxation, hormone secretion, nervous system function, and synergy with other nutrients to function. Flagged as a nutrient of concern for most due to inadequate intakes and long-term proton pump inhibitor medications.

Sources: dairy, dairy alternative milks, wheat and soy flour, molasses, tofu, Brewer's yeast, Brazil nuts, broccoli, cabbage, dark leafy greens, hazelnuts, oysters, sardines, and canned salmon

Phosphorus: Involved with acid-base balance, hormone activation, bone formation, and energy production and storage.

Sources: whole grains, enriched and fortified grain products, seafood, poultry, nuts, seeds, beans, peas, dairy, and meats

Magnesium: Involved in over 300 biochemical reactions, muscle/nerve function, heart rhythm, immune system, and strong bones. Regulates calcium, copper, zinc, potassium, and vitamin D. Flagged as a nutrient of concern due to inadequate intakes.

Sources: avocados, banana, beans and peas, green leafy vegetables, dairy products, nuts and pumpkin seeds, raisins, whole grains, potatoes, and wheat bran

Potassium: Involved in blood pressure regulation, fluid balance, growth and development, carbohydrate metabolism, heart function, muscle contraction, protein formation, and nervous system function. Flagged as a nutrient of concern due to inadequate intakes.

Sources: dairy products, bananas, beans, tomatoes, spinach, prunes, sweet and white potatoes, orange and orange juice, and beet greens

Sodium: Involved with acid-base balance, fluid balance, muscle contraction, blood pressure regulation, and nervous system function. Flagged as a nutrient commonly consumed in excess as compared to the other electrolytes (potassium, magnesium, chloride, calcium, and phosphorous).

Sources: table salt, poultry, baked goods, cheese, deli items, cured meats, snack foods, packaged/convenience/canned foods, soups (you may notice that many foods that are sources of sodium are not the most supportive of health and wellness)

Chloride: Involved with acid-base balance, conversion of food into energy, fluid balance, digestion, and nervous system function.

Sources: celery, lettuce, olives, rye, salt substitutes, seaweeds (e.g., dulse and kelp), tomatoes, table salt, and sea salt

Trace Minerals: Job Duties and Food Sources

Iron: Flagged as a nutrient of concern in young children, pregnant women, and women of child-bearing age. Can also be of concern with poorly planned vegan/vegetarian diets. Involved with energy production, growth and development, immune function, red blood cell formation, reproduction, and wound healing.

Sources: beans and peas, dark green vegetables, enriched and fortified cereals and breads, meats, poultry, prunes and prune juice, raisins, seafood, and whole grains

Chromium: Functions with assisting insulin function, increases fertility, and involved in carbohydrate and fat metabolism. Essential for fetal growth and development.

Sources: Brewer's yeast, whole grains, seafood, green beans, broccoli, prunes, nuts, potatoes, meats, spices (e.g., garlic and cinnamon), basil, turkey, apples, bananas, and grape and orange juices

Copper: An antioxidant involved in bone formation, collagen and connective tissue formation, energy production, hair and skin coloring, and taste sensitivity. Stimulates iron absorption and nervous system function, helps metabolize several fatty acids.

Sources: oysters, seeds, dark leafy vegetables, organ meats, dried legumes, whole grains, nuts, shellfish, lentils, chocolate, cocoa, soybeans, oats, and blackstrap molasses

Zinc: Supports enzymes, the immune system, wound healing, taste/smell, DNA synthesis, and normal growth and development during pregnancy, childhood, and adolescence.

Sources: oysters, red meat, poultry, beans, nuts, seafood, whole grains, fortified breakfast cereals, and dairy

Manganese: Involved with carbohydrate, protein, and cholesterol metabolism, cartilage and bone formation, and wound healing.

Sources: beans, nuts, pineapple, spinach, sweet potato, and whole grains

Molybdenum: Involved with enzyme production.

Sources: beans and peas, nuts, and whole grains

Iodine: Involved with growth and development, metabolism, reproduction, and thyroid hormone production.

Sources: breads and cereals, dairy products, iodized salt, potatoes, seafood, seaweed, and turkey

Selenium: An antioxidant, works with vitamin E, helps with immune function and prostaglandin production.

Sources: Brewer's yeast, wheat germ, liver, butter, cold-water fish, shellfish, garlic, whole grains, sunflower seeds, and Brazil nuts

Water: Job Duties and Sources

Water accounts for about 60 percent of an adult's body weight. Your lean muscle tissue is about 75 percent water, whereas fat tissue is only 25 percent water. Therefore, those with smaller proportions of lean muscle mass, such as females, the elderly, and obese people will have a lower proportion of their total body weight as water. Water literally is the fluid of life. You can go three weeks without food, but only three days without water.

Water has a pretty significant job description. It carries nutrients, removes waste products, and acts as a solvent, a lubricant, and a cushion. Water maintains your blood volume and the structural integrity of large molecules. It's needed for metabolic reactions and helps to regulate your body temperature. Without adequate water your mental and physical performance will be impacted. It is also necessary to keep the kidneys, heart, GI tract, and each body system functioning properly.

It's important to note that your thirst response lags behind the body's need for water so by the time you feel thirsty you're already dehydrated. A good rule of thumb is to aim to drink half of your body weight (or ideal or adjusted body weight if you are obese) in fluid ounces. For example, if you are 150 pounds, then aim for 75 ounces of water per day. Fluid needs increase during illness (e.g., fevers, flu) and strenuous exercise and activity. We lose water as vapor from our lungs as part of the breathing process, in sweat from our skin, and during excretion in urine and feces.

Be aware of the signs of dehydration. Early signs include thirst, weakness, fatigue, dry mouth, flushed skin, decreased urine output, apathy, or impatience. As dehydration worsens, symptoms include headaches, trouble concentrating or focusing, irritability, sleeplessness, increased respirations, and trouble regulating body temperature. Severe dehydration will include such symptoms as dizziness, muscle spasms, exhaustion, loss of balance, delirium, and collapse.

There is such a thing called water intoxication. You may recall over the years hearing about numerous cases of fraternity pledges that unfortunately died from water poisoning as a result of hazing. Drinking 10 to 20 liters of water within a few hours can have disastrous effects on the electrolyte balance in the body and thus cause confusion, convulsions, and even death.

Sources: Drinking water (which actually only provides about one-third of total daily water intakes), other foods and beverages, and your metabolism, which creates water as a by-product as energy-yielding nutrients are broken down.

Debating the merits of different styles of diet is not the goal of this book. The dietary recommendations we will cover later are geared specifically for our target goal of stem cell optimization and activation.

Risk Factors

As you strive to take control over your health, pause for a moment to consider any risk factors that may adversely affect your health. Risk factors are conditions that increase your chance of getting a disease and fall into two categories: modifiable or nonmodifiable.

Examples of nonmodifiable risk factors include age, gender, ethnic background, and family history. Our lifestyle choices are key modifiable factors that influence our overall health, wellness, and susceptibility to disease. Modifiable risk factors include smoking, high blood pressure, insulin resistance, pre-diabetes or diabetes, physical inactivity, being overweight, and high blood cholesterol.

It's no secret that consuming an unhealthy diet is one of the major contributing factors to many diseases, such as type 2 diabetes, cardiovascular disease, dementia, and even certain forms of cancer. We are bombarded daily with sound bites and news reports on the latest research linking specific foods to a health issue or concern. However, statistics continue to show that in the United States poor diet is considered to be the leading cause of death and the third leading cause of Disability-Adjusted Life Year loss, which measures the number of years lost as a result of ill health, disability, or premature death.

Our diets are dramatically impacting and reducing people's life expectancies. With all of the information we possess about diet and nutrition, how much of it is actually being translated from knowledge and being put into practice? Where are we still running into challenges? Let's take a quick look at the status of the Standard American Diet (SAD).

A recent study performed by the Friedman School of Nutrition Science and Policy at Tufts University and the Harvard T. H. Chan School of Public Health looked at the quality of the American diet and the trends in food intake in 44,000 adults from 1999–2016. This study is essentially an 18-year report card on the macronutrient trends in the American diet. The researchers looked at 18 years' worth of data from the National Health and Nutrition Examination Survey (NHANES). The NHANES program is a group of studies using interviews and physical examinations designed to assess the health and nutritional status of adults and children in the United States. When looking at that data, we do see that the macronutrient distribution of Americans' food choices has improved—slightly. Americans are consuming less low-quality carbohydrates and eating whole grains, plant-based proteins, and polyunsaturated fatty acids. However, the improvements are not great enough to counterbalance the amount of diet-related health issues our country faces.

Despite the increased availability of nutrition and diet-related information, unfortunately, this data clearly demonstrates that adults are still eating too many low-quality carbohydrates and more than the recommended daily amount of saturated fat. There was only a 1.23 percent increase in consumption of high-quality carbohydrates; with that increase, high-quality carbs still only account for less than 9 percent of total daily energy. There was a 3.25 percent decrease in low-quality carbohydrate intake due to a decline in consuming added sugars and fruit juice However, low-quality carbohydrates from refined grains, starchy vegetables, and added sugars still account for 42 percent of the typical American's daily calories! The estimated percentage of energy from total protein increased by 0.82 percent, thereby providing about 16.4 percent of daily calories. The increase in protein sources was seen in both animal and plant-based sources. Total fat increased by 1.20 percent, making fat a 33.2 percent contributor to daily caloric intake.

We can see that, although Americans' food choices have improved during this 18-year period, the proportion of energy coming from poor-quality carbohydrates or processed carbohydrates is still too high. Americans' saturated fat intake also continues to be higher than recommended.

It is interesting to see how these trends correlate with changes in nutrition messaging from the government, mainly in the form of the Dietary Guidelines for Americans (DGA). These recommendations have also evolved somewhat over the years.

A Brief Look at the DGA's History

The USDA began issuing dietary recommendations back in 1894 by way of a Farmers' Bulletin, and the first USDA food guide, *Food for Young Children*, was released in 1916. In 1917, *How to Select Foods* was aimed toward the general public. This basic guide was modified over the next few years to provide shopping guidelines based on family size.

In the decades to follow, nutrition information evolved:

- **1941:** Recommended Dietary Allowances (RDAs) were released with specific recommended intakes for calories and nine essential nutrients. They were protein, iron, calcium, vitamins A and D, thiamin, riboflavin, niacin, and ascorbic acid (vitamin C).

- **1943:** USDA released the Basic Seven food guide, outlining a foundational diet that would provide a majority of the RDAs for nutrients, but only a portion of caloric needs.

- **1956:** The Basic Four recommended a minimum number of foods from each of the four food groups: milk, meats, fruits and vegetables, and grain products.

- **1977:** Dietary Goals for the United States: Here we begin to see the emphasis moving from obtaining adequate nutrients to avoiding excessive amounts of food constituents linked to chronic illnesses. The report listed goals for intakes of protein, carbohydrates, fatty acids, cholesterol, sugars, and sodium.

- **1979:** Hassle-Free Guide to a Better Diet, a new food guide, included the basic four food groups but also introduced a fifth food group: "fats, sweets, and alcoholic beverages," with the goal of moderation.

- **1980:** The first edition of Nutrition and Your Health Dietary Guidelines for Americans focused on a variety of foods and not quantities. It included recommendations for maintaining a healthy body weight and moderation with fat, saturated fat, cholesterol, and sodium.

- **From 1980 to present:** The Dietary Guidelines for Americans have been revised and republished every five years.

- **1992:** The Food Guide Pyramid was released. This tool was to be used in conjunction with the dietary guidelines to illustrate how the guidelines could be put into action.

The original dietary guidelines published in 1980 listed the following guidelines:

- Eat a variety of foods.
- Maintain ideal weight.
- Avoid too much fat, saturated fat, and cholesterol.
- Eat foods with adequate starch and fiber.
- Avoid too much sugar.
- Avoid too much sodium.
- If you drink alcohol, do so in moderation.

The current 2015 to 2020 dietary guidelines are:

- Follow a healthy eating pattern across the lifespan.
- Focus on a variety of nutrient-dense foods and the amount of food being consumed.
- Limit calories from added sugars and saturated fats, and reduce sodium.
- Shift to healthier food and beverage choices.
- Support a healthy eating pattern for all.

Even with published guidelines, it is understandable that confusion persists over diet and nutrition. Just turn on the evening news, pick up a newspaper, or scan the front covers of magazines at the grocery checkout. Further compounding the level of confusion is the overwhelming amount of information available online, the majority of which is not evidence-based; or the evidence has been cherry-picked and wordsmithed into a glossy tagline and blog post. It can be challenging for clinicians to stay up to date with the most current body of evidence, so it stands to reason that it can be extremely overwhelming for the average person to make heads or tails of all of the chronically conflicting information we are given regarding our diet.

For example, look at the visual difference between the Food Pyramid and the current MyPlate educational tools. Decades of shaming fats and cholesterol are no longer commonplace among those in the know. Eggs and real butter are back on the menu. We have seen some improvements in the composition and quality as well. So, yes, Americans are gradually decreasing their intake of added sugars and increasing consumption of whole grains, poultry, and nuts.

As scientific evidence has evolved, slowly we've seen a minor revision to the Dietary Guidelines with an increased focus on promotion of the health benefits of good healthy fats and more plant-based sources of proteins. It took some time, but there is also more discussion now about the harmful nature of poor-quality carbohydrates and added sugars. Have you ever seen the documentary film *Fed Up*? If not, it's worth taking a peek. However, I am not a big fan of many of the food "shock-u-mentaries" out there, because they tend to leave viewers overwhelmed, scared, or even more confused.

Aside from government-supplied nutritional advice, we cannot ignore the influence that modern popular diets have had on the shifting trends. For example, note the increasing popularity of Atkins (this one seems to ride a new wave of popularity every ten years or so), paleo/primal/ancestral, low-carbohydrate, ketogenic, plant-based, etc. In fact, a recent systematic review of popular diets found some interesting results that are not in accordance with current recommendations of the 2015 Dietary Guidelines Advisory Committee. The advisory committee reported that diets providing less than 45 percent of daily calories in the form of carbohydrates are not more successful than other diets for long-term weight loss. This category of diets would include Atkins and paleo. However, the 2017 review showed that both the Atkins and paleo diets resulted in substantial long-term weight losses in a number of clinical studies.

How SAD Are We?

Now, let's get back to our report card. There have been decades of guidelines, and we're still facing the same dietary challenges. We may not have gotten a big red "F," but we are far from receiving a passing grade. The small amount of improvement that has been observed in macronutrient composition is a step in the right direction. However, the overall quality of our population's diet did not improve.

We know that a main contributing factor to the declining health in America is overconsumption; we consume more energy than necessary, and that energy sourcing is often from poor-quality carbohydrates, such as refined grains, fruit juice, potatoes, and added sugars in food or in beverages. Saturated fat intake remains above the recommended intake of total calories. As for our protein marks, Americans are relying more heavily on protein sources from animal foods, such as red meat and processed meat, and protein intake from seafood and plant-based sources is still relatively low by comparison.

It is important to note that numerous studies show that the consumption of red meat and processed meats is associated with poorer health. However, a caveat here is there has not been enough research directly comparing the health outcomes in diets relying upon organic, grass-fed, and pastured animal products. We need better research studies to evaluate the quality of the animal-sourced products as compared to conventionally raised animal protein sources.

We must also address the contributing factors of age, education level, race, ethnicity, and socioeconomic status. There is no easy and quick fix to solve this complicated puzzle. However, the report card does serve as a reminder of what is working, what is not working well, and where more targeted education and programming are needed. There's a reason why the standard American diet is referred to as SAD, for it is a sorry state of affairs. We know there's still a lot of room left for improvement. However, that does not mean that we should all sit back and wait as the research, nutrition education, and community programming catches up. The most simple thing that each person can do immediately to change their diet is look at the quality of their choices. By merely starting off by reducing the amount of processed, packaged, and convenience items you eat and replacing them with real, minimally processed whole foods made mostly from plants, you're on the right track. Remember to shop the outer perimeter of the grocery store—that's where most of the live food is. The inner aisles contain many of the SAD items (dead, nutrient-poor food).

Chapter 3

THE HUNGER GAMES

There is an overwhelming abundance of evidenced-based research illustrating how profound the role of diet is in terms of human health. This is not a newsflash to any of us (or at least it shouldn't be in this day and age), and we covered the most current findings, looking at the SAD diet, in Chapter 2. Although this book is not intended to be a primer on human nutrition and diet therapy, we do need to cover some additional scientific facts in order to appreciate fully the impact that food choices can have on our topic at hand: stem cells. Keep that in mind; the topics we discuss are based upon the impact on stem cells, and your stem cells are dramatically affected by your diet!

A Body in Balance

Let's take a moment here to pause and quickly look at the idea of homeostasis. The word "homeostasis" comes from the Greek words for "same" and "steady." When we use the term homeostasis in a biological sense, we are referring to processes that organisms employ to keep things stable, or the action to return to a stable condition. Obtaining and maintaining homeostasis is necessary for survival. Examples of homeostasis in the human body include regulation of body temperature, blood glucose levels, oxygenation, electrolytes, and fluids. Stem cells hold the golden key to helping your tissues maintain homeostasis by doing their jobs of self-renewal and differentiation. But are there things that you are doing that could be changing the locks?

While we're on the topic of homeostasis and the Greeks' influence on medicine, let's pay homage to Hippocrates, the Greek physician, born in 460 BC, who is considered the father of modern medicine. In fact, the oath that new doctors take is called the Hippocratic Oath, and one of Hippocrates' most notable quotes is "Let food be thy medicine and medicine be thy food." Another one of his brilliant observations is that "All disease begins in the gut." Even more than 2,000 years ago, the digestive system was recognized as being a key player in whole-body health or diseases. Sadly, with all of our current knowledge and technological advances, many fail to recognize the role one's digestive health can play in a person's overall health. Many consider the heart or the brain to be the most important factor, but I would argue that your gastrointestinal system is the most important.

The GI Tract Command Center

Your gastrointestinal (GI) tract, or digestive system, is responsible for far more than simply digesting, absorbing, and eliminating the foods you eat. The surface area of one's intestinal lining is approximately 4,305 square feet (400 square meters) long. Within this system also resides your gut flora, which comprises your individual microbiome. The GI tract also houses roughly 70 percent of your body's immune system, serving as a protective barrier against microorganisms and antigens (a molecule capable of causing an immune response in the body). Antigens influence the body's reactions to foods and, therefore, play an important role in the development of food sensitivities, inflammatory conditions, and chronic diseases. The GI tract is also the production source for approximately two-thirds of your body's hormones and neurotransmitters. Personally, I consider the GI tract to be the command center for the rest of the body. If this system is not functioning properly, there is no way for the body to be in homeostasis. For some, it may not be blatantly obvious when there is an issue with how well their GI tract is functioning. This is where we might want to look at things a bit more simplistically.

A Fine-Tuned Machine

To a certain extent, the human body functions like a machine. Our parts and systems are interwoven, intended to work together to maintain life. In my private practice, I will frequently ask a client to envision what their dream vehicle would be and what they would expect that vehicle to be capable of doing. What kind of performance are they looking forward to getting out of that vehicle? What kind of maintenance will the vehicle need? What would be the quality of the fuel and oil they would use in that vehicle? Imagine now a high-end performance vehicle, and the manufacturer suggests using premium or 93 octane fuel and the best-quality synthetic blend oil. What would happen to the performance of that vehicle if lesser-grade gasoline and motor oil were used? Will that vehicle perform as expected? What will happen to the fuel economy? Would the gas mileage be poor, thus requiring more frequent fill-ups? Your body does run very similarly to a high-performance vehicle, and your system's performance is affected greatly by the quality of the food (aka fuel and oil) that the engine is given. Hippocrates recognized this more than 2 millennia ago.

The health of your GI tract has great influence over how well homeostasis is being maintained throughout the body. If stem cells hold the key to helping our tissues maintain homeostasis through self-renewal and differentiation, then our GI tract can literally be the open doorway accepting of the stem cell key or become a complicated padlock requiring the help of a lock-smith. This is where your diet is a determining factor in holding the right key to your dream vehicle. Ask yourself, do I want to be behind the wheel of a finely tuned machine, or am I okay with driving through life in an old jalopy?

Calorie Wars

It's difficult to have a discussion about diet without the oblig-atory question about caloric goals. Although the focus of this book is not weight loss, obesity statistics alone dictate that we should spend some time discussing it. There is a strong like-lihood that weight loss or maintenance is part of your overall wellness goals, whether you are trying to lose fifty pounds or the last five vanity pounds. Additionally, our caloric needs continue to decrease as our age increases, and evidence suggests that a degree of caloric restriction is best for longevity and anti-aging. So, this is not a topic to be ignored.

How often have you heard, "If you want to lose weight you just need to eat less and move more"? Or, "A pound of fat is equal to 3,500 calories, so if you want to lose a pound of fat you need to create a calorie deficit of 3,500 calories." Calories, calories, calories. So, let's talk about calorie wars.

If you are like most of us, at some point you have used either an app or an online tool to calculate your estimated energy needs. These equations use your height, weight, age, and gender to estimate your caloric needs. It may seem like a bit of alphabet soup when you're looking at the different names of these measurements of daily calories. Basal metabolic rate (BMR), resting metabolic rate (RMR), basal energy expenditure (BEE), resting energy expenditure (REE). What do they all mean? Are they all the same?

While these terms are often used interchangeably, there are some subtle differences between them. Both BMR and RMR are used to estimate the number of calories you would burn over a 24-hour period at rest. Therefore, they are used to calculate the minimum number of calories or energy that your body needs to keep functioning. Remember homeostasis? Your body needs a certain level of fuel in order to keep your body temperature, you're breathing and respiration, and your brain, heart, and organ systems functioning properly.

While we have mathematical equations that allow us to estimate caloric needs, both BMR and RMR can be measured more precisely in a clinical setting using direct or indirect calorimetry. This is where the differences between both measurements are seen. Of the two, BMR—also known as basal energy expenditure (BEE)—is more strict when being measured in a clinical setting. The test is generally conducted after the individual has slept in a darkened room for at least eight hours, and the measurement is taken immediately upon waking. The individual has also fasted for at least 12 hours and is lying down, relaxed during the measurement to ensure accuracy. When RMR—also referred to as resting energy expenditure (REE)—is performed in a clinical setting, the individual is lying back and rested, but this test can be done at any point during the day, typically after only having a three- to four-hour fasting period. This method also does not require the person to sleep in a facility or to have had at least eight hours of sleep before having the measurement taken.

The main difference between BMR and RMR is that RMR also takes into account the minimum number of calories that would be burned while eating or just doing light activities of daily living. Truth be told, though, in the scientific literature the difference between RMR and BMR is usually less than 10 percent of total calories. Regardless of which equation you use, you should be aware of some factors that can affect your results.

Factors That Can Influence Your BMR

- Resting metabolic rate slows down as we age.

- As your weight decreases, BMR also decreases.

- Environmental temperature has a role in BMR, but not as much of a role as you may be hoping for.

- Genetics might have a bigger role than you may realize, but you will need to have a nutritionally focused genetic panel done to find out exactly how big.

- Muscle is more metabolically active tissue than fat. More muscle mass means an increase in your metabolic rate.

- BMR is a bit of a chauvinist; it is usually higher in men than in women.

- Illness can raise your RMR as your body fights an infection.

- Micronutrient deficiencies can decrease metabolic rate.

- Movement and exercise can increase your metabolic rate.

Common Equations for Determining Caloric Needs

The Original Harris-Benedict Equation

Men BMR = 66.4730 + (13.7516 x weight in kg) + (5.0033 x height in cm) - (6.7550 x age in years)

Women BMR = 655.0955 + (9.5634 x weight in kg) + (1.8496 x height in cm) - (4.6756 x age in years)

The Revised Harris-Benedict Equation

Men BMR = 88.362 + (13.397 x weight in kg) + (4.799 x height in cm) - (5.677 x age in years)

Women BMR = 447.593 + (9.247 x weight in kg) + (3.098 x height in cm) - (4.330 x age in years)

The Mifflin-St Jeor Equation

Men BMR = (10 x weight in kg) + (6.25 x height in cm) - (5 x age in years) + 5 (measured in Kcal/day)

Women BMR = (10 x weight in kg) + (6.25 x height in cm) - (5 x age in years) - 161 (measured in Kcal/day)

The Katch-McArdle Formula (Resting Daily Energy Expenditure)

BMR = 370 + (21.6 x LBM) - LBM = lean body mass in Kg

The Cunningham Formula (RMR)

BMR = 500 + (22 x LBM) - LBM = lean body mass in Kg

Now that you have an estimate of your daily caloric needs, what will you do with that information? If you are following traditional weight-loss dogma and are aiming to lose fat, you would be finding a way to reduce your daily calories to lose 1 pound of fat for every 3,500-calorie deficit you recorded. Maybe you're considering using a combination of caloric restriction in conjunction with increased energy expenditure through movement or exercise. We've been told ad nauseam that weight loss is purely an equation—a teeter-totter of sorts. This see-saw has the total calories consumed by a person sitting on one side and calories out (calories expended or burned through metabolic processes, heat, exercise, and life) sitting on the opposite side. If you want to lose weight, you need to expend more energy than you consume. So, where did this calories-in-calories-out philosophy originate? It boils down to physics. The calories-in-calories-out (CICO) mantra is based upon the first Law of Thermodynamics, which states that energy cannot be created or destroyed—it can only be changed. The problem here is that a narrow view only focusing on the thermodynamics in a manner that stresses CICO alone doesn't allow then for paying enough attention to human physiology, especially where digestion, absorption, utilization, assimilation, and transport of nutrients is concerned, and influences metabolism.

Let's stop and think for a moment as to how successful the calories-in-calories-out philosophy has been in terms of weight loss overall. Does caloric restriction lead to weight loss? Yes, a caloric deficit will lead to weight loss, but isn't the goal of weight management long-term success? If weight management was purely just a teeter-totter equation of balance, would the weight-loss industry be the multibillion-dollar industry that it is today? Would we have so many dieting failures? Wouldn't it be very simple for people to lose weight if they just cut back some calories and exercised a little bit more? That's what most doctors seem to tell their patients to do. Simple, right? I mean, come on, we're talking about simple math here, right?

After 25 years of practice as a dietitian, I can attest that the CICO theory alone does not work for the long haul. Long-term weight-loss success is usually defined as results that last 12 months or longer. CICO is definitely part of the conversation when it comes to long-term weight loss, but it is not the major tipping point. Remember the old adage that the definition of insanity is doing the same thing over and over and expecting a different result? If you've done the calorie-counting game over and over, it's time to stop banging your head against that wall and move on. (Though, actually, banging your head against a wall is thought to burn 150 calories per hour.) You need to drill down to what works best for *your* body.

Simply put, not all calories are created equal! The source and the quality of your calories matter. Entire volumes of work and research have been devoted to debating the *quality* question, but quality trumps quantity in my book. Remember our discussion on the quality of the fuel source? What are you putting into your tank? If you put cheap gas into a high-performance engine, that engine is going to require more fuel in a shorter period of time.

Also, while the machine will burn through the cheap fuel, the performance and efficiency of the engine will suffer greatly than if given better-quality fuel. Remember better fuel, better overall performance. Therefore, in the debate around weight management do we focus on total calories or should we dive deeper and look at the quality of those calories and follow the physiological response that our bodies have to our fuel sources? We cannot ignore how a fuel source will affect ingestion, digestion, absorption, assimilation, egestion, and ultimately, utilization of the nutrients.

The CICO camp tends to look at energy in terms of deposits and withdrawals. Imagine if you will that your body has a bank vault where your energy stores are kept. If your calorie intake exceeds your calorie output, theory would dictate that your body will package and store those excess calories and make a deposit into your fat vault. If only things were that simple. What often gets overlooked in the CICO philosophy is the fact that, historically, reducing total calories came in conjunction with lower-fat, higher-carbohydrate intake. How has that low-fat, higher-carbohydrate (but usually insufficient in fiber), calorically restricted program worked for people over the years? A prime example of its failure is the research that was done on the contestants for the TV weight-loss program *The Biggest Loser*.

Losing in More Ways Than One and on National Television

A study published in 2016 looked at fourteen former contestants; it followed them during their thirty weeks on the ranch, and then for six years afterward, and monitored their weight as well as markers of metabolic function and body composition. During their time on the ranch the contestants lost, on average, more than a hundred pounds each, which is considered a tremendous feat and a great success. But what was the long-lasting cost of that rapid dramatic weight loss? Bear in mind that during the program the contestants' average caloric intake was about 1,200 calories per day, and they engaged in intense physical activity for at least ninety minutes per day, six days a week.

Unfortunately, the results for many were short-lived. These contestants ended up being a prime example of a phenomenon called "metabolic adaptation," or *adaptive thermogenesis*. Remember how we established that your resting metabolic rate will go down in conjunction with a decrease in your body weight? When metabolic adaptation occurs, that change and decrease in metabolic rate often occurs in a greater proportion than what would generally be expected based upon one's measured body composition, meaning their muscle mass compared to fat mass. This process is thought to be a protective response: When your body is "thinking" that you are starving, it goes into starvation mode. You may be making a conscious effort to reduce calories, but your body is going to respond to the decrease in available fuel in a different way.

Think of caloric restriction in terms of a caloric lay-off of sorts. Essentially, calories can be likened to a workforce (remember the construction workers). Thus, when you reduce your caloric workers, say by 300 to 500 calories per day, you are still asking the body to produce and maintain its daily processes. When there's been a workforce reduction—a lay-off of calories—the remaining workers need to become more efficient to keep production at the same level. In the face of caloric restriction, your body learns to become more efficient by adapting its metabolic rate. That, unfortunately, results in your metabolic rate becoming lessened or slowed. It is expected to rebound and increase when body weight again increases and caloric intake returns to what could be viewed as a normal amount. In theory, the metabolism would respond in kind by returning to a "normal" level.

The cruel irony with the *Biggest Loser* research group was that this did not occur. Their weight increased and they did regain some muscle mass, which theoretically should have allowed for some increase in the resting metabolic rate. But overall on average, each contestant's basal metabolic rate was approximately 500 calories less than where it should have been, based upon the contestants' height, weight, age, and body composition. To add insult to injury, it was also observed that the participants had hormonal imbalances, not only in the thyroid hormone but also the hormones regulating hunger and satiety. Leptin is your satiety hormone and ghrelin is your hunger hormone. Typically, leptin and your resting metabolic rate have a direct relationship, meaning they increase and decrease together. If your weight falls, your resting metabolic rate and leptin levels fall. As your weight increases, in theory, your leptin and resting metabolic rate would both go up. However, in *The Biggest Loser* participants, while their leptin levels did rise in accordance with their regains, unfortunately, their metabolisms did not bounce back.

Leptin and ghrelin are hormones necessary to regulate appetite, which ultimately influences one's body weight. It's a cycle: We get hungry, we eat, we get full, we stop eating. Leptin is the hormone responsible for telling us that we are satisfied, and ghrelin is the hormone that triggers your hunger. While they are both secreting peripherally in the body, they end up in the brain and signal the hypothalamus.

Leptin is released mainly by your fat cells, but also from the stomach, heart, placenta, and skeletal muscle. Leptin *reduces* hunger. Ghrelin is released mainly by the lining of the stomach. Ghrelin *raises* hunger. Think ghrelin: growl! Each of these hormones will respond to how well-fed someone is. It's intended to be a directional relationship—the more fat mass you have, the more leptin you make. Therefore, theoretically, more fat = more leptin = less hunger. Conversely for leaner persons, less fat mass = less leptin = more hunger.

The quandary, though, for many with higher body fat is that they often report high levels of hunger. They may have more than an ample supply of leptin, but somehow the brain isn't listening. The appetite stays high, but the metabolism doesn't increase to correspond with leptin levels, and the brain thinks the body is starving. What the heck is going on? How are the signals getting so crossed? These folks may be stuck in the vicious cycle of leptin resistance. Leptin resistance ironically shares signaling pathways to insulin resistance, which is also often seen in those with excess body fat mass. In both instances, the excessive amounts of each hormone being produced has resulted in the brain ignoring the message. Were *The Biggest Loser* contestants doomed from the start following the kind of regimen they followed? Clearly the program was not the key to long-term success. Let's circle back to the CICO camp to finish looking at physics and physiology.

Are You the Key Master? I Am the Gatekeeper

Let's explore why CICO is only one portion of the puzzle. Bear with me here; this will all make sense when we add the stem cell puzzle pieces later. Bring back the image of your bank vault and your key ring. In a perfect world, CICO would be a simplistic way to manage weight. In actuality, our bodies are far more complex, with a system of checks and balances that regulate all of our body's processes.

There is a system to regulate how we burn our calories, when we burn, and when we store. A major key holder in this system is the anabolic hormone insulin. Produced by your pancreas, insulin holds a fairly sizeable key on your key ring. This hormone is responsible for controlling the metabolism of carbohydrates, lipids, and protein. It holds the key to direct the availability of fuel sources in both fasting and fed states. When you're in a fed state, insulin signals energy utilization and uptake. The insulin is released in response to feeding and has numerous job duties. It will result in energy deposits in your bank vault in the form of glycogen and fat. It will also decrease the amount of glucose produced by the liver while also unlocking the doorway for entry of glucose in muscle, adipose (fat), and other body tissues.

Just as insulin signals the fed state, glucagon sounds the bell for the fasted state. Glucagon will be triggered when insulin secretion decreases and blood glucose levels drop. Glucagon stimulates glycogen breakdown, calling for a withdrawal from the fat vault so it can be used for energy. By doing their job properly in fasting or feeding, insulin and glucagon are responsible for maintaining homeostasis of glucose levels in the bloodstream.

But what does insulin have to do with quality of my food choices? Say you have two plates of food that are equivalent in calories, such as a plate of brownies versus a grilled chicken and vegetable dish. Your body's response to your food choice would be different, particularly in terms of the amount of insulin that would be released in response to the constituents of the meal. The argument here is, if we only focus on calories, we lose sight of the hormonal response that is occurring.

A traditional weight-loss plan would see you cutting calories and fat but consuming a high percentage of your total calories from carbohydrates. Therefore, despite lower calories, your insulin levels would remain high, especially if those carbohydrate calories were from higher glycemic foods. If insulin is high, your body is in storage mode. If you're trying to lose weight, you want to be in withdrawal mode, taking fat out of the bank vault, not setting the stage to be making even more deposits, especially when you're really hungry because you've cut your calories.

Your diet choice is now going to work against you, making it even harder to hold true over the long haul. You're essentially trying to unlock the door to success with the wrong key. You've now hopped on the same roller coaster that many CICO alumni have. You're hungry, maybe even "hangry." At some point in the near future, you will hit a plateau and face the decision either to move more or eat even less. At this crossroads, most people throw in the towel and feel like a failure. Even if they don't immediately go back to their old habits, at this point if they go above the new threshold that was created in response to a caloric deficit, the weight will come back on, and somehow a few extra pounds get thrown in for good measure. You can thank your slower metabolism for the spiteful insult. Whether your goal is weight loss or stem cell activation, you need to break that yo-yo cycle and preserve your metabolism.

Call the Locksmith

Now, let's look at things through a different lens. For all those who believe in the CICO as the be-all-end-all key to success, my question is this: How is that working for the millions of Americans struggling with their weight? Instead, shift focus away from reducing calories and aim more toward reducing insulin. Diet strategies that manipulate intakes of total carbohydrates, such as low-carb, modified ketogenic, ketogenic, cyclical keto/carb cycling, and fasting regimens can have a positive influence on the degree of insulin secretion, meaning they result in reducing the amount of insulin released when fasting and feeding.

With a focus on insulin instead of total calories, you now have a key available to unlock the vault and allow your stored energy to be withdrawn and spent (utilized). Will this result in overall fewer total calories than what you had been consuming? In some instances, yes, especially if you were using fasting methods (more on that later). However, it's not just about the total calories, remember? It's about the sources of the calories, and these styles of diet result in less insulin being secreted. The added bonus here is that research shows, unlike in CICO, your metabolic rate does not take a beating. Your appetite may, in fact, decrease too (alongside your waistline). It's a good day when you and your body are both on the same side rather than at opposing ends.

Chapter 4

SLOWING DOWN THE CLOCK—OPTIMIZING YOUR STEM CELLS

If you're scratching your head and wondering what all this has to do with your stem cells, your patience is about to be rewarded. I challenge you to keep an open mind and remember that, at the end of the day, we need to find a balance between what might be optimal and what is most realistic.

Diet's Impact on the Job Performance of Stem Cells

We covered how the link between diet, health, and disease is well-established. Diet can be used for disease prevention as well as to help with treatment. Volumes of scientific literature support how dietary restriction promotes metabolic and cellular changes that affect oxidative damage and inflammation, optimize energy metabolism, and enhance cellular protection.

The quality of your diet directly affects the overall nutrient density of your intake and, in turn, the availability of nutrients needed in sufficient supply to meet your body's demand to perform its tasks. Dietary nutrients play an important role in the maintenance of tissues and adult stem cells in diverse tissues. For example, vitamin C can regulate how hematopoietic stem cells function, through ten-eleven translocation (TET2) enzymes and a low level of dietary vitamin D can compromise the function of stem cells in the intestine. To put it in simpler terms, nutrients tell our cells what to do.

Even the way you prepare and combine the ingredients in foods can influence health and wellness (we'll cover this in more detail in Chapter 6). Dietary composition and calorie levels are key factors affecting how well we age and what age-related diseases we face. We should never underestimate the power that diet has over our health. Science has shown us just how responsive stem cells are to changes in our bodies. Stem cells respond to these shifts and help to organize and transform tissues. Recognizing that certain cancers are thought to develop from these transformed stem cells and tissues, we are reminded of how strong the connection between our diet, our stem cell function, and cancer risk is.

Whether you are an athlete who is developing her muscles, a pregnant mother with a developing fetus, or a person struggling with the ravages of aging, the right foods can help increase the amount and performance of your stem cells and their ability to regenerate your body.

We can avoid some risks for our stem cells by controlling our blood sugar and reducing our exposure to air pollution, tobacco, and alcohol. But some other risks are more difficult to avoid. Aging, for example, is constantly reducing our ability to regenerate.

Slowing the Sands of Time: Anti-Aging Interventions

Aging is an inevitable part of life. The quest to age gracefully, slow the process, or even halt it is the focus of billions of dollars spent annually. From a scientific view, what we have to look forward to in the aging process is functional decline, a steady increase of a variety of chronic diseases, and ultimately, death. Is it any wonder we continually search for ways to improve and extend our lives? Evolutionary theory includes a process called natural selection, a set of checks and balances intended to provide protection of a species by ensuring the "survival of the fittest" and, thus, the creation of healthy offspring. Aging and death, also part of the evolutionary process, is theorized to be necessary to prevent overpopulation and to continue ensuring that only the healthiest of DNA gets passed on to the next generation.

In our search for the Fountain of Youth and tools to help us age gracefully, if we are going to extend our lifespan, how do we ensure from a cellular level that we are supporting the body's need to carry out cellular functions that support longevity effectively? It's not enough to just protect our body from the effects of aging but rather empowering our bodies with the tools to help repair, regenerate, or even replace at the cellular level, the main construction site.

Getting old itself puts us at higher risk for numerous diseases, and in the spirit of self-preservation, wouldn't it be wise to be actively proactive and take the initial steps to slow the aging process rather than being reactive after damage has already occurred and illness has set in?

Simply put, aging is a reduction in our body's ability to regenerate—our stem cells slacking off on the job. The amount of stem cells we possess and their abilities diminish with age. It is estimated that the percentage of people aged 65 years and older in the United States will account for 19.3 percent of the population by 2030. Though the percentage of the aging population will continue to grow, health span and lifespan are not the same. Despite all of the advances and successes made in science and medicine, the fact is that the rate of new diseases is skyrocketing. Noncommunicable diseases, such as cancer, heart disease, stroke, diabetes, obesity, and neurodegenerative diseases, are the major health threats to people around the world. Sadly, health span is not pacing neck and neck with lifespan. The World Health Organization (WHO) maintains that age continues to be the biggest risk factor for all major life-threatening disorders. As lifespan increases, the number of people facing age-related diseases is expected to nearly double in the next 20 years.

Complicating matters is the prevalence of weight-related issues. The percentage of the adult population in the United States who are obese or overweight has risen over 70 percent. One out of every three adults in the US has hypertension. Both obesity and hypertension represent major risk factors for stroke and cardiovascular disease. Although weight loss and an increase in physical activity are generally prescribed to avoid such age-associated diseases, only a small percentage of people have the discipline to change their lifestyles accordingly. The prevalence of age-related pathologies represents major psychological and social impediments as well as an economic burden that urgently needs appropriate interventions.

What can we do to manipulate the aging process? Are there any tools at our disposal that do not require spending tens of thousands of dollars? Can the fountain of youth really be found in your refrigerator? The answer to all three questions is, "Yes." Numerous recent studies have shown the benefit that the style of diet and exercise programs can have on your senescence (we'll get into this deeper in Chapter 6). Low-calorie diets combined with activity have been proven to counteract the aging process. From a biological standpoint, it really means drilling down to a few cellular processes to achieve the most effective impact on aging. These include nutrient signaling, mitochondrial efficiency (the ratio in the amount of ATP generated per unit of oxygen consumed), proteostasis (protein homeostasis), and autophagy (literally mean self-eating, the body's way of clearing out older or damaged cells, we'll discuss this in more detail later).

Anytime there is a mention of reversing the signs of aging or slowing the aging process or aging gracefully, you are bound to raise some interest and attention. It's not so much of a question of when we will age but more of how and why do we age? If our stem cells potentially hold the key to our immortality, why must we age? This sounds like a rhetorical question, but from a biological standpoint, we know that continual maintenance and repair of all of our cells would require a large supply and demand for energy, and from an evolutionary standpoint immortality may prevent adaptation and survival of the fittest.

When we narrow the playing field and focus specifically on dietary regimens aimed at healthy aging, it's important to understand how the process works. Once we understand the underlying mechanisms involved, the next step is actually taking that knowledge and putting it into practice. The latter can sometimes prove hardest for people. Here we turn again to the scientific literature to provide a basis of evidence-based research. When using a critical eye and requiring that strict criteria are met, only three lifestyle interventions lead to the "fountain of youth." These are exercise, caloric restriction, and fasting regimens. Let's look at each one individually and highlight the pros and the cons.

Exercise

From an anti-aging and longevity standpoint, we know that exercise has been shown to provide benefits in avoiding cardiovascular disease, diabetes, osteoporosis, sarcopenia, and depression, as well as prolonging the level of independence in the elderly. Exercise also has documented benefits in reducing our risk of morbidity and mortality. Moderate or low levels of exercise, even in the absence of weight loss, still have been shown to provide a positive benefit. One area where exercise shines is that it is the only known treatment for the prevention or reversal of sarcopenia, a disease of age-related muscle strength and function loss.

There has been some interesting research looking at the combination of exercise and caloric restrictions for health promotion. Alternate-day fasting in conjunction with exercise has been shown to provide greater benefit for muscle mass over exercise by itself. In normal-weight subjects, exercise combined with caloric restriction actually showed better effects on insulin sensitivity as well as decreasing levels of C-reactive protein, which is a marker of inflammation.

Despite all its benefits at improving our overall quality of life, regular exercise has not been shown to extend our lifespan. But hands down, a regular exercise regimen will help you to age more healthfully and, ultimately, more gracefully. Plus, we know that exercise does induce autophagy, which is on the stem cell activation key ring!

Auto-What?

The term autophagy comes from Greek, meaning "self-eating," and is the process that breaks down and cleans out damaged cells in order to regenerate newer, healthier cells. It's the body's way of recycling. Both fasting and caloric restriction are strong inducers of autophagy. In a feast-or-famine scenario, this process is an efficient strategy to maintain life during famine until resources again become available. Autophagy works to ensure that sufficient energy levels are maintained while also working to eliminate damaged cellular material. As we age and/or when more fat accumulates, our natural ability to induce autophagy decreases. Though excess fat suppresses this process, burning of fat for primary fuel (lipolysis and then ketosis) seems to activate it.

Caloric Restriction (CR)

To eat or not to eat? That is the main question when it comes to stem cells and diet. When evaluating all of the available science that looks at dietary interventions to influence and optimize stem cells, one theme is seen consistently, time and time again: Caloric restriction has been shown in the literature to preserve the function of stem cells.

You may be thinking, "Wait a minute—we just spent the better part of Chapter 3 debating the merits of caloric restriction!" Indeed we did. However, now as we dig into the science regarding caloric restriction in regard to stem cells, we will see how the research unfolds for us, providing a plan that combines caloric restriction with specifics on the timing of the restriction, frequency, duration, and nutrient density. There are a few theories on how caloric restriction can lead to a longer life as well as activation of your stem cells. Truth be told, much of the research to date is from mouse studies, but there are a handful of human studies.

We've spent a lot of time talking about this particular intervention. The obvious pros include reduction in body fat, blood pressure, and resting heart rate, and lipid panel improvements. The cons include risk of malnutrition, which then can contribute to neurological issues, fertility, sex drive, problems with wound healing, changes to menses, osteopenia and osteoporosis, as well as decreased immune strength.

Ideally, in the research, a caloric restriction of around 15 percent does provide benefits in aging. The process by which caloric restriction exerts its benefits as an anti-aging mechanism is the reduction in release of growth factors, such as growth hormone insulin and insulin-like growth factor 1 (IGF-1). Each of these is associated with speeding up the aging process as well as increasing mortality rates.

According to the 2015–2020 Dietary Guidelines, adult women need roughly 1,600–2,400 calories per day and adult men need approximately 2,000–3,000 calories per day. More sedentary adults, male or female, should opt for the lower end of the recommended range while those leading active lifestyles can lean toward the higher end.

Our calorie needs also decrease as we age. Sadly, most people underestimate their daily intake by at least 1,000 calories. If you have never logged your food, it may be an eye-opening exercise for you to get a truer picture of your intake. Be honest, no one will be looking over your shoulder passing judgment. But if it passes your lips, it needs to be logged.

When using any food-tracking tools a few things to consider: Make sure you are entering the amount you actually consumed, not the standard portion size listed for a food. Also, be leery of entries made by other users as they are less likely to be accurate. If you're having trouble locating information on a food item, check out the USDA's Food Central website at https://fdc.nal .usda.gov.

Once you've assessed what your average intake should be as compared to what it is in actuality, you can begin decreasing total calories by 15 percent and then working your way down until you are at 15 percent less than your recommended targeted daily calories.

It's important to remember that caloric restriction without focus on quality of those calories can negate some of its beneficial effects. There is evidence showing that a healthy diet alone allows for a longer life span in animal models without needing additional benefit from caloric restriction; therefore, the quality of your diet may end up sparing you the need to follow a calorie-restricted diet. Caloric restriction influences numerous processes in the aging body; these include the transcriptome (collection of all the gene readouts present in a cell), hormonal status, oxidative stress, markers of inflammation, mitochondrial function (these guys are the powerhouse of your cells), and the all-important homeostatic control over glucose.

As for those who are firmly ingrained in the high-protein camp, unfortunately, the research is stacking against them in the aging department. There is an ongoing debate about protein goals for older adults and for healthy aging. However, the evidence focusing specifically on longevity tends to suggest a protein restriction is necessary if you are seeking anti-aging benefits. The restriction of protein allows for depletion of IGF-1.

The caveat when mentioning protein restriction is, it really boils down to consuming adequate protein based on age and body weight. The Recommended Dietary Allowance (RDA) is 0.8 grams (.02 ounces) of protein per kilogram (2.2 pounds) of body weight. This would typically supply about 10 percent of one's total daily calories.

However, the average American consumes around 16 percent of their total calories from protein. The typical American diet provides large amounts of protein by nutritional requirement standards. Keeping protein intake more in line with recommendations based on need will seem very much like a restriction to the vast majority. But don't forget that there is no one-size-fits-all (or most), so in determining a target protein intake when a goal is anti-aging and longevity, we also need to consider factors such as current health status, kidney function, current lean muscle mass, activity level, and immune status.

The Dark Side of Caloric Restriction

Despite some of its documented benefits, there are some concerns with the long-term use of CR. CR leads to loss of fat-free mass (lean muscle mass), thereby slowing metabolic rate and predisposing individuals to weight gain. Let me say it again for emphasis—CR triggers a metabolic adaptation that reduces 24-hour energy expenditure beyond the expected for reduction in metabolic mass (*The Biggest Loser* gang dealt with this). Long-term compliance to CR is notoriously low.

Fasting Regimens

It seems almost counterproductive to deprive ourselves of nutrition from food. However, fasting has profound effects on how our cells behave. Fasting has been practiced for millennia and has been seen in some form in just about every culture and religion around the globe. Recent studies have shed light on its role in adaptive cellular responses that reduce oxidative damage and inflammation, optimize energy metabolism, and boost cellular protection.

In lower eukaryotes (any cell or organism that possesses a clearly defined nucleus), chronic fasting extends longevity, in part by reprogramming metabolic and stress-resistance pathways. In rodents, intermittent or periodic fasting protects against diabetes, cancers, heart disease, and neurodegeneration. Fasting has the potential to delay aging, activate stem cells, and help prevent and treat diseases while minimizing the side effects caused by chronic dietary interventions.

In humans, fasting has been shown to be beneficial in improving lipids (LDL cholesterol, triglycerides) and in treating:

- Obesity

- Hypertension

- Dysglycemia/blood sugar control issues (insulin resistance, type 1 diabetes, type 2 diabetes)

- Immunosenescence (the decline in the immune response as we age)

- Autoimmune diseases, such as rheumatoid arthritis and multiple sclerosis

- Neurodegenerative disorders, including Alzheimer's disease, Parkinson's disease, and ALS

Fasting regimens are contraindicated in those who are underweight or pregnant, or are in certain disease states. It should also go without saying that fasting is encouraged to be done in association with an overall healthy diet.

Mechanisms behind the Magic of Fasting

What happens in the body when we fast? Remember our discussion in Chapter 3 about making deposits and withdrawals from our energy vault? When you fast, your body experiences a set of metabolic changes in order to meet your energy needs. Once you have burned through your stores of glycogen, the hormone glucagon and a process called gluconeogenesis will be activated.

Gluconeogenesis literally means "to create glucose" and is the process by which glucose is made from non-sugar sources, such as lactate, pyruvate, and glucogenic amino acids. Both lactate and pyruvate are molecules in the body that can be converted into glucose. They are both also involved in numerous biochemical pathways and the presence or absence of oxygen can impact the pathway direction (remember high school science terms like aerobic, anaerobic, and the Kreb's Cycle?).

Additionally, during fasting your body will convert fat into fatty acids, which can then be absorbed by the blood.

The metabolic switch that gets turned on during fasting allows your body to move from burning glucose as a primary fuel source to using fatty acids and ketones. This switch can be flipped in as little as eight to twelve hours of fasting. Contrary to previous beliefs that ketones were not an efficient or even healthy fuel source, current research illustrates how ketones are your body's and brain's preferred fuel source during fasting and during extended periods of exercising, even if you are not currently practicing a fasting regimen. The benefit here is that ketones are a cleaner fuel source than glucose, carbohydrates, or protein, because ketones produce far fewer metabolic disruptors (molecules that can damage cells).

Based on research evidence, it appears that fasting regimens have an advantage over long-term or permanent caloric restriction. Fasting may help you to avoid those negative effects and the dark side of caloric restriction. Fasting regimens do not cause the loss of lean muscle tissue as is typically seen in caloric restriction. There's a big difference between being in ketosis and ketoacidosis, the latter of which is a life-threatening medical emergency usually associated with diabetes.

The change in cellular behavior in response to fasting provides keys to improvement and maintenance of health. Recent studies illustrate how fasting for 24 hours increases stem cell activity in mice. These mice were fasted for 24 hours and then researchers obtained stem cells from the lining of their intestines. Their stem cells were then grown in a culture and analyzed to measure their activity. Researchers found that in the group of mice that had been fasted, the regenerative ability of their stem cells doubled as compared to the mice that had not been fasting.

Thankfully, it's not just lab mice where we see positive changes and stem cell activity in response to fasting. Multiple studies on humans have shown how fasting anywhere from twenty-four to seventy-two hours triggers stem cell regeneration that ultimately rejuvenates the body's immune system. Fasting not only forces the body to use stores of glucose, fat, and ketones, but also causes a breakdown in a significant number of white blood cells. This reduction of white blood cells stimulates changes that activate stem cell–based regeneration of new immune system cells.

The key is prolonged fasting (not just fasting overnight for your annual blood tests). We'll define the styles of fasting in a bit.

Though we can't expect what is seen in mouse models to translate into expectations in human studies, studies have shown that rats following an alternate-day fasting regimen live up to 83 percent longer than rats fed a normal diet. Mouse models have also shown that life expectancy was significantly extended in groups who were on a regimen of being fasted for a 24-hour period every four days.[4]

Other trials of fasting and mice demonstrated fat mice who were fed a high-fat diet in a time-restricted feeding protocol ended up having lower markers of inflammation and no evidence of fatty liver, and were slimmer as compared to mice who were fed an equivalent number of calories but without restrictions on time and access to those calories. How does this apply to humans? Let's get science-y again.

When food is scarce—whether because of famine or conscious fasting—your body is going to trigger a few mechanisms. These mechanisms aim to conserve energy and do so by decreasing cellular growth pathways. One main focus is on the nutrient-sensing pathways. Nutrient sensing is a vital part of life. When food is in abundance, the nutrient-sensing pathways set in motion mechanisms for anabolism (building up) and storage. On the flipside, in times of food scarcity, they trigger homeostatic operations, such as the movement of internal stores by actions such as autophagy.

The body achieves this by controlling key nutrient-sensing pathways, such as IGF-1, m-TOR (mammalian target of rapamycin is a protein that plays a role in control of some cell functions like

---

4   Longo and Mattson, "Fasting: Molecular Mechanisms and Clinical Applications," 181–192.

cell division and survival), and PKA (protein kinase A is a family of enzymes responsible for regulating a cell's activity and can influence protein, sugar, glycogen, and fat metabolism). All three of these are also linked to promote aging. In many disease states, the nutrient-sensing pathways become unregulated.

If we follow the logic of these pathways, increasing them speeds up aging, and decreasing them slows down aging. By regulating these pathways, the downstream effect results in some incredible benefits:

- Cell maintenance and protection are increased.

- Inflammation is decreased.

- Autophagy is triggered

- Stress-resistance responses are improved.

Research completed at USC's Longevity Institute demonstrates how a fasting-mimicking diet (FMD) blocks the activity of the major pro-aging genes, like IGF-1, TOR, and PKA. In the process of blocking those pathways, you've now allowed for the promotion of pathways that results in regeneration, which leads to rejuvenation, and when you're rejuvenated, you're impacting the longevity of your cells. When those pro-aging pathways are inhibited, your cells in tissues enter into a mode that activates certain enzymes triggering protection and repair. Secondly, damaged cells and cellular components are destroyed, which then paves the way for your stem cells to be activated and unleash their renewing properties.

Let's look at the history of human frequency of food intake over the centuries. We have evolved from consuming one meal per day to eating two meals then three meals, to consuming three meals plus a snack, and finally to the common current practice of three meals plus multiple snacks per day. Evolutionary history provides the evidence that we are, in fact, built to fast. Our ancestors relied on the hunt and the harvest. Our bodies possess the ability to survive during periods of hunger, which is essentially fasting. Compared to present-day eating habits, we have come a long way from the days of feast or famine.

Styles of Fasting Defined

Fasting is complete absence of food intake. There are a few popular styles of fasting. When you are considering beginning a fasting regimen, I strongly encourage you to work with a knowledgeable, licensed clinician or functional medicine–trained dietitian/nutritionist to help you determine which of the following styles of fasting would be best for you.

Prolonged Fasting

Prolonged fasting refers to at least two and usually three or more consecutive fasting days, which can be repeated periodically. These are water-only fasts. The truth of the matter here is that, despite the benefits of water-only fasts, they typically have a 90 percent dropout rate after 24 hours. Losses of 5 to 15 percent of lean muscle have been seen in five-day water fasts. For some, there are also concerns about the change in intestinal permeability with water-only fasts. This is definitely one style of fast that should absolutely be done under medical supervision, for there are numerous pros and cons to be considered at the individual level.

Intermittent Fasting

Intermittent fasting (IF) eliminates or greatly reduces daily intake of food/calories intermittently (usually every other day or every two to three days).

Time-restricted feeding (TRF) is a form of intermittent fasting that means alternating a feeding window with a fasting window of time.

- 14:10: Fast for fourteen hours straight (overnight/sleep is included in this) and then consume all meals/snacks in a ten-hour window. For example, have breakfast at 6 a.m. and your last meal by 4 p.m. and then nothing else until 6 a.m. the next day.

- 16:8: Fast for sixteen hours straight (overnight/sleep is included in this) and then consume all meals/snacks in an eight-hour window. For example, have breakfast at 8 a.m. and your last meal by 4 p.m. and then nothing else until 8 a.m. the next day.

Alternate-Day Fasting

Usually, alternate-day fasting (ADF) refers to alternation of a day of feeding and a day of either water-only fasting or a very-low-calorie diet.

- Eat Stop Eat means fasting for a full 24-hour period once or twice per week (not on consecutive days). On non-fast days, you would consume a healthy, high-quality diet.

- 5:2: During two non-consecutive days of the week, you restrict your total calories to approximately 300 to 500 for the day. On non-fast days, you would consume a healthy, high-quality diet.

Fasting-Mimicking Diets (FMDs)

Fasting-mimicking diets (FMDs) are specifically designed combinations of food so that the composition of macronutrients and micronutrients is formulated to trigger responses such as reduced glucose and insulin-like growth factor 1 level, and increased ketone bodies, while maximizing caloric intake.

The FMD style of fasting aims to provide 800 to 1,100 calories per day. Your body thinks it is being fasted, but you are actually still eating. FMD employs a plant-based diet that is low in protein, carbohydrates, sugars, and high fat. The specific ratios of macronutrients and micronutrients used in FMD trick your body, allowing fasting mechanisms to kick in while you are still being fed to an extent. When you are following the FMD protocol, the diet is followed for five consecutive days a month for three consecutive months.

FMD is the subject of Dr. Valter Longo's best-selling book *The Longevity Diet*. An FMD program, ProLon, is commercially available through a company called L-Nutra. Those interested in using FMD can either follow the detailed specific food formula in Longo's book or opt for the ProLon kits. I have been a TRF'er myself for the past five years, and ProLon is the FMD tool I use and referenced in the introduction pages of this book.

Note that I am *not* on L-Nutra's payroll. I use the product because I believe in it and have seen firsthand the effects it can have. After completing my first three rounds, I now do a "maintenance" round every three or four months. Doing FMD on your own is also entirely feasible; however, I have found that when fasting for five days, the last things I wanted to do were planning, prepping, portioning, and cooking. The kit makes it much easier, which increases compliance and, ultimately, success.

In the scientific literature, FMD is said to cause a systemic anti-inflammatory effect and specific suppression of autoimmune cells, whereas the refeeding period stimulates hematopoietic cells to generate naïve cells to replace the immune cells eliminated.[5] These naïve T cells have differentiated in bone marrow and while considered to be mature cells, they have yet to be exposed to any antigen, thus the term "naïve." FMD also promotes tissue-specific stem cells that repair the damaged sites. FMD boosts levels of circulating stem cells in the blood and stimulates autophagy.

After five days of FMD, stem cells were increased by 800 percent. Additionally, research on FMD has shown that using this intervention reduces body weight, abdominal fat, blood pressure, blood fats, markers of inflammation, and IGF-1 (a tumor marker), while preserving lean body mass and maintaining healthy blood glucose levels.

FMD was also shown to keep IGF-1 at healthy levels, and even five to eight days after resuming a normal diet, research participants still had a 15 percent reduction in the pro-aging hormone.[6] For those dealing with hypertension, fasting has been shown to be the most effective way to lower blood pressure. In fact, trials of FMD have shown that even four months after completing the three cycles of the protocol, participants have sustained benefits, including maintenance of 60 percent of the weight loss.[7]

5   Cheng, Villani, Buono et al., "Fasting-Mimicking Diet Promotes Ngn3-Driven Cell Regeneration to Reverse Diabetes," 775–788.

6   Brandhorst, Choi, Wei et al., "A Periodic Diet That Mimics Fasting Promotes Multi-System Regeneration, Enhanced Cognitive Performance, and Healthspan," 86–99.

7   Choi, Lee, and Longo, "Nutrition and Fasting Mimicking Diets in the Prevention and Treatment of Autoimmune Diseases and Immunosenescence," 4–12.

How Does It Work?

When you use fasting as an intervention, the body will transition through some distinct phases. The first three are induction days, followed by a mode activating cellular-protection mechanisms and priming stem cells and DNA, followed by the goal of the program: rejuvenation and regeneration.

If you are following a five-day FMD program, here is an example of what is going on behind the scenes on a day-to-day basis:

- **Day 1:** You begin to enter the fasting state and so begins the transition to start optimizing your cellular processes.

- **Day 2:** You have now switched to fat-burning mode using ketones for energy. The process of autophagy has also begun turning your body into a cellular recycling center.

- **Day 3:** You are most likely in full ketosis, and cellular housecleaning is in full swing.

- **Day 4:** Stem cell regeneration begins. Essentially, it takes you two days to get into the full fasting state and then two days to clean house.

- **Day 5:** There is a significant increase in the number of circulating stem cells that your body can now tap into and harness for their regenerative capabilities.

The power of these stem cells doesn't stop after day five; the research on FMD suggests that the regeneration and rejuvenation stage continues past day ten, five days after you have stopped fasting.

SYSTEMIC BENEFITS OF FASTING

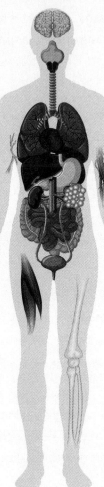

Heart/Cardiovascular System

- Resting heart rate decreases
- Blood pressure is reduced
- Stress resistance improves
- Parasympathetic tone (the part of the autonomic nervous system that slows heart rate, increases digestive and glandular activity, and relaxes the sphincter muscles) increases

Digestive System/ Liver & Intestines

- Markers of oxidative stress decrease
- Liver glycogen is depleted
- Ketones are produced
- Insulin sensitivity increases
- Accumulation of lipids are reduced
- Intestinal motility improves
- Intestinal inflammation is reduced

Muscle/Skeletal System

- Insulin sensitivity increases
- Inflammation decreases
- Endurance and efficiency improve

Brain/Neurological System

- Cognition improves
- Neurotrophic factors (substances that control rapid cell growth and differentiation in the nervous system) are produced
- Synaptic plasticity (ability of synapses to strengthen or weaken over time, depending on increases or decreases in their activity)
- Mitochondrial biogenesis (the growth and division of preexisting mitochondria)
- Resistance to disease and injury improves

Blood/Circulatory System

- Ketone levels increase
- Adiponectin levels increase
- Glucose, leptin, and insulin levels all decrease
- Inflammatory cytokines are reduced
- Markers of oxidative stress decrease

Adipose (Fat) Tissue/ Integumentary System

- Leptin production is reduced
- Inflammation decreases
- Lipolysis occurs (the breaking down of fats to be used for energy)

How Safe Is Long-Term Fasting?

Whether you opt for fasting or caloric restriction, it's important to be aware that neither should be done unsupervised for extended periods of time. Be mindful of changes to your body composition; you are not just experiencing losses of body fat, but also precious lean muscle mass.

Micronutrient insufficiency and clinical deficiency are also of concern. You may be questioning the need for dietary supplements during the time you are manipulating your diet for the purpose of stem cell optimization. The irony here is that the use of supplements may actually backfire on you: You may end up supporting the health of the cell that you want to die so your body can clean house and trigger the generation of new healthy cells.

Some facts to bear in mind when fasting:

- Stay hydrated. You should be drinking at least 64 ounces of water per day.

- Be cautious with operating vehicles and heavy machinery until you know how fasting is going to affect you.

- Avoid strenuous exercise and swimming while fasting.

- Avoid exposure to extreme temperatures—this can include the use of saunas, spas, hot tubs, and cryotherapy tanks.

- While fasting you may experience weakness, headache, caffeine withdrawal, muscle pain, dry mouth, and memory impairment.

We have discussed the current body of research illustrating how caloric restriction and fasting regimens exert positive effects on stem cell function. The debate over the use of a high-fat or ketogenic diet rages on; this is because, historically, the scientific literature shows that high-fat diets tend to have negative effects on stem cells by impairing their function or even creating opportunities for tumor formation. However, recently published research from MIT scientists sheds some light on how a high-fat diet can actually improve the function of intestinal stem cells. This study showed that high levels of ketone bodies (which become present in fasting or high-fat ketogenic diets that trigger ketosis) help the intestine to keep a large pool of adult stem cells. These stem cells are critically important for keeping the intestinal lining healthy.[8]

Have you heard the terms intestinal permeability, increased intestinal permeability, and leaky gut? Yeah, that's a subject for another book entirely, but we will explore it a bit more in Chapter 5!

These MIT researchers also discovered that intestinal stem cells produced curiously high levels of ketone bodies, even without a high-fat diet. Their study also sheds light on how ketones impact signaling pathways, such as Notch—a pathway that has been shown to help regulate stem cell differentiation. This research can help us to understand better how ketone bodies can instruct an intestinal stem cell and thereby determine its fate. Further research is needed to help us better understand how high-fat diets and ketones can help to boost intestinal stem cells for the purpose of regeneration. Research has also established the link between high-fat diets and some intestinal cancers that arise from intestinal stem cells.

---

8   Cheng et al., "Ketone Body Signaling Mediates Intestinal Stem Cell Homeostasis and Adaptation to Diet."

Chapter 5

WHAT'S MY GUT GOT TO DO WITH THIS?

Actually, your gut has a lot to do with stem cells. Without a healthy gut, you're decreasing your opportunity to activate your miracle-working stem cells. The frightening fact is that poor gut health runs rampant in our modern society. Thirty-five visits to a doctor for every 100 people are for digestive concerns. In the US, 20 percent of the population suffers with gastroesophageal reflux disease, and irritable bowel syndrome (IBS) affects about 10 to 15 percent of the population. Nearly three million Americans have been diagnosed with autoimmune inflammatory bowel diseases like Crohn's disease and ulcerative colitis. It's estimated that 1 in every 133 people has celiac disease, the autoimmune disease where consumption of gluten (a protein found in wheat, barley, and rye) causes damage to the lining of the small intestine.

I haven't even touched upon the less common GI issues either. One alarming area is the prevalence of small intestine bacterial overgrowth (SIBO) and small intestine fungal overgrowth. While exact statistics for these conditions are hard to come by, the estimates for IBS patients who also have SIBO range from 30 percent up to a whopping 80 percent. We are a population of people dealing with chronic GI complaints, and many people have been lulled into thinking that's just life and they just have to live with these symptoms.

You've probably been hearing the term microbiome being tossed around—even in body wash commercials. The truth is, every tissue of the body is thought to have its own microbiome; our tissues are not sterile. But that doesn't mean this is a bad thing. Humans are teeming with microbes. In fact, every time you get on the scale, three to five pounds of your body weight is microbes. We have trillions of them that live on and inside us. The cells of microbes outnumber our own cells ten to one. Often when you hear the term microbiome without a reference to a specific region, the term is most likely referencing the GI tract.

Why are our microbes so important? They have their own set of job duties in the body and without them, healthfulness would be impossible. Microbes help us with digestion, nutrient provision, and absorption. They provide a line of immune defense merely by occupying space that may have been desirable to an invader, give a boost to our immune system, and protect us from autoimmune diseases. Evidence exists to support their role in epigenetics, weight management, stress tolerance, detoxification, and specific conditions such as rheumatoid arthritis, autism spectrum disorder, fibromyalgia, myalgic encephalomyelitis (formerly known as chronic fatigue syndrome), and even mental health disorders.

Increasing evidence links changes in the balance of the microbes in GI microbiome to the aging of stem cells. These changes can trigger dysfunctions of metabolism and abnormal activation of the immune system, and they can encourage epigenetic instability of stem cells. Factors that can contribute to the change in balance (also known as dysbiosis) are hormones, inflammation, and the immune system. A key to the health of your microbiome is having a diverse population (think of the diversity training you may have gone through at work). There is health, vitality, and strength in communities where there is diversity in cultures, and this holds true for our microbiome too.

Back in Chapter 2, we described the GI tract's complicated job description, and the ways in which it is responsible for far more than simply digesting, absorbing, and eliminating the foods we eat. The surface area of your intestinal lining is approximately 4,305 square feet long and requires about 40 percent of your body's energy expenditure. What a wonder this organ is! Incredibly, it fits nice and compact in our mid-sections. As discussed previously, I consider the GI tract to be the epicenter of the body. Poor GI health will eventually lead to declining health in other body systems. There is not a single health condition or disease that does not in some way link back to the gut. One of the main reasons for this is a major job duty of the GI tract is sheltering approximately 70 percent of your body's immune system.

Your Diet, Gut, and Immune Health

In order to fully appreciate the role the gut plays in regard to stem cells, let's dig a bit deeper into the relationship between your diet, gut, and immune health. Most Americans are well aware that a drive-through diet is probably not in the best interest of their waistlines and annual check-ups. But how many people recognize the role their SAD/drive-through/fast-food diets can have on their immune system? How often are we bombarded with ads, especially in the winter months, for products aimed to "boost our immune system"? Maybe the immune boost we need is to bypass the local fast food joint.

We've already established that Americans chronically overconsume calories and are also undernourished. Calorically dense foods are not always the most nutrient dense. The SAD is usually high in salt, poor-quality saturated fat, and sugar. This disparity between caloric density versus nutrient density is well-established when looking at the SAD's impact on obesity and chronic illnesses like heart disease, cancers, diabetes, and kidney disease.

As Hippocrates stated, "all disease begins in the gut," and the majority of our immune system lives in our gut, so it's only logical to make the connection that a SAD eating habit will eventually impact the strength of our immune systems. But how exactly? Well, there are quite a few ways that this domino effect gets underway. Follow along with me:

• The SAD leads to obesity and an increase in fat cells (adipocytes). Adipocytes release pro-inflammatory substances including interleukin-1 (IL-1), IL-6, and tumor necrosis factor. The overproduction of these pro-inflammatory cytokines can cause the immune system to slow down its response times (think the boy who cried wolf) so when there truly is an issue your immune response may be delayed.

• Obese persons usually have fewer white blood cells to fight infection and reduced phagocytosis ability (the ability to engulf another cell to destroy it). They also tend to have higher levels of leptin in the blood. Leptin is known to stimulate natural killer cells, activates the transcription factor STAT3 (which controls cell responses to cytokines and growth factors), and reduces the anti-inflammatory regulatory T cells (Treg) cells (Treg cells suppress the immune response and help prevent auto-immunity; they help maintain immune homeostasis).

- A diet high in sugar reduces white blood cell phagocytosis and increases inflammatory cytokine markers. This significantly reduces the vigor of the immune system. It can also lead to dysbiosis.

- A diet high in salt can increase inflammation and can make autoimmune conditions worse.

Circling back to debates on poor-quality, high-fat, and nutritionally deficient diets in relation to stem cells, these diets have been shown to negatively affect the diversity of the microbiome, and thus can contribute to the aging of intestinal stem cells. This downward spiral begins when poor-quality saturated fats cause multiple immune-related concerns:

- Activates numerous pro-inflammatory pathways and increases IL-17 production and macrophage activation (macrophages are white blood cells that locate and eats foreign invaders).

- Certain receptor signaling can go awry when exposed to saturated fats in too great of amounts or too often (think wires getting crossed and fried).

- Increases gut inflammation and reduces gut barrier function. An inflamed gut plus a weakened gut barrier equals whole body ill-health waiting to happen.

- Causes dysbiosis.

- Trans fats contribute to increased IL-6 and C-reactive protein (CRP) levels—both are markers of inflammation.

- High omega-6 intakes increase inflammation and activate the immune system and can cause dysbiosis.

By now, I hope you're beginning to reflect on your own perceived level of gut health. There are more reasons to love your gut. Additional functions of the intestinal lining are to protect against fluid and electrolyte loss, while allowing molecules, such as nutrients from your food, to be exchanged from within and outside of the GI tract. This exchange of molecules occurs between the tight junctions of the cells that line the surface of your gut, the enterocytes. These cells function as the gatekeepers, determining what should pass across the gut lining and into your body.

Leaky Gut

The gut lining is a pretty hot topic these days, and for good reason. You may have heard or seen the term "leaky gut." Leaky gut may seem to some like an alternative medicine term; however, the more clinical term of "increased intestinal permeability" is the subject of an ever-growing number of evidence-based research studies and is slowly changing the way conventional providers are looking at disease treatments and management. Evidence-based literature has linked increased intestinal permeability to a variety of chronic illnesses, with a particular focus on its role in autoimmune diseases such as rheumatoid arthritis, celiac disease, Crohn's disease, atopic dermatitis, thyroid disease, and type 1 diabetes.

Your gut lining is meant to be selectively permeable. How then does this process go awry and result in a leaky gut? Think of your GI tract like a screen door. In good conditions, the holes in the screen are selectively permeable; they keep things on the appropriate side of the door—either inside or outside. A leaky gut is like a screen door where the holes in the screen have been widened; its integrity has been weakened by any number of factors, and thus, items that are not intended to begin passing through. The leaky screen of your GI tract becomes weakened by factors such as an imbalance of your gut bacteria, poor diet, or use of antibiotics and other gut-irritating medications. The resulting leaky gut lining sets the stage for protein fragments and bacteria to pass out of the GI tract where they do not belong. These particle escapees are viewed as foreign bodies and as antigens when discovered outside the GI tract. Thus, your immune system is stimulated, antibodies are produced, and the inflammatory cycle begins.

Impact on Stem Cells

Let's follow how this cycle affects our stem cells. Dysbiosis causes an increase in gut permeability and changes the number of by-products (metabolites) produced by the microbes. These metabolites in turn have a negative influence on stem cells' metabolism because of activation of pro-inflammatory cytokines in the immune system and can also exert negative effects on DNA and methylation. Methylation refers to the transfer of or addition of a methyl group between molecules. It's a process of critical importance in the body and ultimately can impact each body system.

The downward spiral of pathways that are triggered can lead to erroneous differentiation of stem cells and overuse of stem cells. This causes a loss of tissue homeostasis and aging. To make matters worse, this process can cause more susceptibility to bacteria or virus-mediated tissues, damages which then call for more stem cells to come to the rescue for tissue repair. This vicious cycle can exhaust your stem cell pool and speed up the aging process.

Giving Your Gut a Tune-Up

People of any age can have leaky gut syndrome. Those taking pain medications, antibiotics, oral contraceptives, or steroids, or who have heartburn or reflux can be at higher risk from the syndrome, whether they've been diagnosed with it or not. People with digestive problems (with or without symptoms) will probably have an underlying leaky gut condition, especially with 8 percent of all Americans having chronic digestive diseases, 6 percent having acute digestive episodes, 43 percent having intermittent digestive issues, and 70 percent reporting having digestive-related symptoms or diseases. People who routinely use large amounts of alcohol and caffeine, and those who eat a diet that is high in refined carbohydrates and chemical food additives are at higher risk. Significant toxic exposure from sources like pathogens (bacteria, viruses, fungi, and parasites) or from chemicals and heavy metals in the environment (or even your old mercury-based dental fillings) can also be risk factors. Those of us who have autoimmune diseases are more likely to have an underlying gut permeability problem as well.

Is it any wonder that the vast majority of us can benefit from a gut health overhaul? One caveat here, if you are suffering with moderate to severe GI symptoms, you should seek the consult of a gastroenterologist and a GI-trained functional dietitian nutritionist to help navigate the steps to improving your gut health. The steps listed next are intended for those who have been living the standard rat-race lifestyle with poor diet, high stress, lack of proper sleep, overuse of antibiotics, etc. You know who you are! Food is information, to your genes, to your cells, and especially, to your stem cells.

The Five R's

In functional nutrition we look at a five-step process, often referred to as "the Five R's," for helping to improve the health of your GI tract. These five steps are:

1. Remove

2. Replace

3. Reinoculate

4. Repair

5. Rebalance

Remove: This process usually begins by removing the foods to which you are sensitive, intolerant, or allergic. You will also want to remove poor quality, processed foods, and refrain from the overconsumption of alcohol. Additionally, look for ways to remove chronic stress and stressors to your GI tract, such as toxins, chemicals, and environmental stressors like pollutants.

Do you use pain medications often? These can cause damage to your gut lining. Are you using other medications such as birth control, steroids, or medication for heartburn or reflux (even the over-the-counter ones)? If so, you may want to work with a functional nutrition provider for education on how to safely address gut health with these medications on board. A functional nutrition provider may also use an elimination diet to help determine what foods may be causing GI symptoms. The goal is to reduce your intake of foods that can trigger systemic reactions in order to reduce inflammation, lower the allergenic load, and provide the gut with a dietary base to allow for restoration. A functional nutrition provider also assesses for pathogenic microflora (bacteria, fungi, parasites) and then use a combination of diet and supportive supplements to eradicate any offending bugs.

Replace: The goal here is providing replacement of or support for digestive factors that may be inadequate or lacking. These factors may be in short supply due to your current diet, health history, diseases, the aging process, medication use, or other factors. Common causes of maldigestion include inadequate mastication (not chewing properly or thoroughly), insufficient hydrochloric acid, insufficient intestinal brush border enzymes, decreased stimulation of the pancreas, insufficient pancreatic enzymes, and insufficient bile acids.

Replacement would include things such as digestive enzymes, hydrochloric acid, pancreatic enzymes, and bile salts. This is where Dr. Google is not a substitute for a consult with a knowledgeable licensed provider to determine personalized interventions based on your unique set of circumstances.

Commonly used interventions may include any combination of the following: Betaine HCL tablets (350–3500 mg) taken with protein-containing meals, consuming umeboshi plums, use of digestive enzymes with acid pH range, use of Swedish/digestive bitters, gentian root, and apple cider vinegar. Don't discount the role of lifestyle factors: Reduce your stress, increase your exercise, and get good-quality sleep. You also want to make sure you are consuming adequate fiber to support GI function, transit, and elimination (aim for at least 25 grams of fiber per day).

Reinoculate: The focus at this step is supportive reintroduction of beneficial GI microflora (prebiotics, probiotics, synbiotics) to achieve a more desirable balance to the intestinal microbiome. You can help this process along by literally feeding your gut foods that contain probiotics, or a clinician may also choose a targeted supplement that contains the "good" GI bacteria like bifidobacteria strains, lactobacillus strains, and *Saccharomyces boulardii*. Fiber is important here because it is the food that the beneficial bacteria like to eat—these are often referred to as prebiotics. Consider prebiotic fibers as the fertilizer for the probiotics. Inulin, fructooligosaccharides, and soluble fibers are helpful to feed your gut.

Foods that help this process include (organic preferred):

Asparagus	Green tea
Bananas	Jerusalem artichokes
Barley	Leeks
Burdock root	Legumes
Chicory	Oats
Chinese chives	Onions
Cultured and fermented foods. Cultured dairy, non-dairy kefir, yogurt, cultured vegetables, miso, and tempeh	Organic non-GMO soybeans
	Peas
	Raw honey
Eggplant	Sugar maple
Flax	Whole fruits
Garlic	Whole wheat

Remember, many antibiotics do not discriminate, they kill both good and bad bacteria. If you need to use an antibiotic, probiotics either from supplements or food are often necessary to help restore a balanced gut flora. If you choose to use a supplement, be sure to take it either two hours before or two hours after your dose of antibiotic.

Repair: The aim of this step is providing the nutritional support for healing and regeneration of the GI mucosa. This becomes the anti-inflammatory foundation for your diet moving forward.

It begins with avoiding the items in the "replace" step and adding foods such as bone broth, steamed vegetables, and mucus-forming foods such as:

licorice tea	okra
marshmallow root tea	slippery elm tea

Personalized interventions from a clinician may include a combination of the following supportive supplements:

arginine	pantothenic acid
carotenoids	phosphatidylcholine, slippery elm, DGL licorice, and marshmallow root (mucosal support)
colostrum	
curcumin	
glutamine	quercetin
fish oil	vitamins A, C, D, and E
lactoferrin	whey immunoglobulins
lactoperoxidase	zinc

Rebalance: This step requires close attention to your lifestyle choices. Sleep quantity, exercise habits, and stress can all affect the health and healing of your GI tract. This step is often the tipping point for many and can be the key to healing (and then supporting stem cell activation) or the key to unraveling all your efforts if this step is not made a priority. Practices to consider are:

- Scheduling self-care time and relaxation
- Mindful eating and better food choices
- Heart rate variability/biofeedback
- Yoga, meditation, prayer, breathing, or other centering practices

- Psychotherapy

The bottom line is that leaky gut affects your stem cells. So if this is something that you suspect that you'll be struggling with, rebalancing your gut microbiota and working to restore gut permeability must be made a priority in order to optimize your stem cells.

Chapter 6

NEXT STEPS—KEYS TO YOUR SUCCESS

By now you should have a good understanding of fasting, macronutrients, micronutrients, and ways to ensure optimal gut health. Bear in mind that we have spent much of this book highlighting how fasting is a key tool for optimizing and activating of your stem cells. While fasting helps support biological processes, over the millennia it has served as part of the evolutionary process. Throughout the ages humans have encountered periods of starvation. There's a reason why the phrase "feast or famine" exists. Fasting can literally be one of a simplest yet most incredibly powerful tools that you can use to stimulate positive changes in your body. It may also have a great impact on your wallet as you decrease the need for doctor appointments, copays, and prescription medications.

How do you take all of the information you've learned thus far and apply it in practice when choosing our foods? If fasting stimulates your stem cells, how can your daily diet keep them healthy and decrease the factors that cause the need to trigger them in the first place? The main answer here goes back to keeping homeostasis, and that requires keeping inflammation and all inflammatory processes we covered under control. Inflammation is a major root cause for degrees of unwellness.

Remove the Roadblocks

Within your grasp is the ability to harness the power of your stem cells through food. Show your stem cells some love with the choices you make each day. In Chapter 5, we dug deep into the science behind gut health—the barometer for whole-body health. Empower your stem cells by choosing to remove the barriers to their optimal function. You can literally keep them on the job by removing their occupational hazards. These hazards include:

Environmental toxins. Limit your exposure to environmental toxins such as air pollution and tobacco as they reduce the number of stem cells in your body that are available for regeneration and repair. Toxins will affect your stem cells. Be mindful of factors such as the quality of the air you breathe and the water you drink. A wonderful resource to help you research these topics further and to narrow down by geography is the Environmental Working Group. Check out their homepage at www.ewg.org.

Dietary sugar. Control your blood sugar and reduce or eliminate added sugar in your diet. Hands-down, sugar is one of biggest offenders working against your stem cells. Much research has shown how this nutrient contributes to aging rapidly and premature death because of its impact on your genetic expression. A diet high in sugar will speed up the aging process while slowing down the factors and enzymes that are intended to protect our bodies from damage, oxidative aging, and *inflammaging* (chronic low-grade inflammation during aging).

Low-quality foods. Improve the quality of what you put into your body; it's the only house you truly get to live in, so take care of it. We've had much discussion in previous chapters on how quality trumps quantity. One of the biggest barriers many of my patients come back with is the argument about organic food being more expensive. There is a sign in my office with the quote "You can either pay the farmer now or pay the doctor later." How I wish most doctors gave out prescriptions for the *farmacy* instead of the pharmacy.

The analogy that I use concerning choosing organic over non-organic foods is to look to simple economics and investment strategies. The term ROI means return on investment. While choosing organic foods may cost a bit more each trip to the grocery store, it's making an investment in your health. You reap returns on this small investment by way of improved health and wellness. But the best investments always have long-term returns. Your weekly investment in organic foods will not only yield short-term rewards but much greater yields over the long haul.

Your risks for chronic diet-related diseases will be decreased, your quality of life will improve, you'll lose less time from work and play due to illness, and you will most likely have a decreased need for doctor's visits and medications. With so many of us dealing with increasing health care costs, high deductible plans, donut holes, etc., doesn't it seem more logical to opt for a prevention plan that includes focusing on your food as part of the prescriptive intervention? Imagine less copays and better-tasting foods.

The power to activate your own stem cells resides within your own kitchen. You don't need special training in the culinary arts nor do you need upscale, boutique grocery stores. A few simple foundational truths can be your basic guide.

With food as medicine, you put healthy in your body in order to get healthy out! There's so much power behind choosing real foods over the pharmacy. In terms of stem cells, food can be the biggest key to unlocking the regenerative power within your own personal reservoir of stem cells. They are just waiting for you to tap into them to help restore your health and vitality.

> *"You can't expect to look like a million bucks when you eat from the dollar menu."*
> —Unknown

Don't forget that quality is paramount and can either enhance the activity of your stem cells or contribute to their demise, which ultimately renders them powerless. Another quote in my office reads, "When you see the Golden Arches, the Pearly Gates are usually not too far behind." Recall our discussion on dietary choices and immune health in Chapter 5.

Poorer-quality foods to consume less of or even avoid entirely are: highly processed snack foods, sugar-laden beverages, refined (white) grains, refined sugar, fried foods, foods high in saturated and trans fats, and high-glycemic foods such as white potatoes. If a food label has more than five ingredients or if sugar is in the first three ingredients, or if you can't pronounce the ingredients, put it back on the shelf and walk away. If you need a PhD in chemistry and a lab to create the food you are considering eating, put it back on the shelf and run away.

While I've made the argument for quality food—organic, locally grown, pesticide free, non-GMO—I recognize that you may need to enter this pool slowly. One consumer-friendly tool is the EWG's Shopping Guides (yes, there's even an app for that). Visit www.ewg.org site and download the "Clean Fifteen" and "Dirty Dozen" lists. As the names imply, the Clean Fifteen consists of the top produce items with the least amount of pesticides and residues in the edible portion. While conversely, the Dirty Dozen are the produce items with the highest amounts of pesticides and residues.

The Clean Fifteen list is a good place to begin funneling your budget for organic food. Begin by committing to buy organic only versions of those items. Check these lists every so often for updates and seasonal changes. In addition:

- Develop an appreciation for real, whole, minimally processed food. You'd be surprised just how amazingly delicious real food is. Explore all your senses and taste buds beyond just sweet and salty.

- Food is intended to nourish the mind, body, and spirit. It's much more than macros and micros. It serves to bind us socially, mentally, physically. Practice gratitude for the nourishing properties of food and for those who made that meal possible for you.

- Food is information to your cells and stem cells.

Your food choices are going to be critical in regulating your health and wellness. Stem cells respond to signals from their environment; your diet and the nutrient composition of your diet provide cues that will influence and alter not only the function but also the activity of your stem cells. Make daily choices to include the foods that have been shown to be anti-inflammatory. Using those anti-inflammatory properties they in turn will help increase the levels of stem cells circulating in your body naturally.

These include foods rich in polyphenols and antioxidants, such as blueberries, green tea, pomegranates, goji berries, and spirulina. Choose the bright colors of the rainbow, especially the deeper, darker blues, red, and purples. These anti-inflammatory foods are often rich in phytonutrients. The natural compounds are nature's little powerhouses in plants and have numerous benefits to our health. Countless studies have illustrated how eating more plant foods translates into reduced risk of chronic diseases such as diabetes, heart disease, and cancer.

Phytonutrients not only help us but the plants in which they are found. They protect the plant from pests and environmental stressors. For us, they provide numerous benefits. Phytonutrients help to stimulate enzymes that help us get rid of toxins, give a boost to the immune system, promote healthy hormone metabolism (like estrogen), enhance cardiovascular health, and hasten the death of cancer cells.

Foods That Support Stem Cells

You may need to adjust these based on your known tolerances. The most common foods to remove for an elimination diet are wheat, eggs, corn, soy, nuts, peanuts, and dairy.

Proteins

Vary your sources and be sure to include plant-based proteins each day. Intake will vary based on your individual needs.

Plant-Based (organic, non-GMO preferred)

dried beans

dried peas

lentils

spirulina

soy (casein free): tofu, tempeh, edamame, soy milk, soy yogurt

Animal-Based (organic, grass fed, hormone free, antibiotic free preferred)

beef	elk
bison	lamb
chicken	turkey
duck	venison
eggs (pastured)	

Fish (wild caught preferred)

Canned fish should be in water and labeled as mercury and BPA free. Aim for more fish rich in omega-3 fats, such as wild Alaskan salmon, herring, sardines, and black cod.

Other fish to consider:

grouper	red snapper
haddock	sea bass
halibut	trout
mackerel	tuna
mahi mahi	walleye

Dairy and Dairy Alternatives (choose unsweetened and plain)

almond milk

coconut milk

dairy (organic, grass-fed, or even raw if you have access to it): cow, sheep, or goat's milk, cheeses, yogurt, and kefir. Fat free or even low fat is not necessary.

Carbohydrates (organic, non-GMO preferred)

Non-Starchy Vegetables

Eat the rainbow. Local, seasonal is best. Aim for at least six to eight (½ cup cooked, 1 cup raw) servings per day to maximize phytonutrient intake regardless of your caloric goals!

artichoke	mushrooms
arugula	mustard greens
asparagus	onions
beets	okra
bell peppers	parsnips
bok choy	peas
broccoli	peppers (all)
Brussels sprouts	pumpkin
cabbage	radish
carrots	romaine lettuce
cauliflower	sauerkraut
celery	seaweed
collards	spinach
cucumbers	squashes
eggplant	tomatoes
garlic	turnip greens
green beans	watercress
kale	

Starchy Vegetables and Whole Grains

Use in moderation.

beans (pulls double duty as a protein and carb)

brown rice

potatoes

quinoa

sweet potatoes

whole and cracked grains

whole oats

wild rice

Fruits

Eat the rainbow. Local, seasonal is best. Eat your fruits, try not to drink them. Avoid dried fruits, aim for tennis-ball size portions.

Choose lower-glycemic index fruits more often:

all berries

apples

lemons

limes

oranges

pears

Choose higher-glycemic index fruits in moderation:

apricots

bananas

cantaloupes

cherries

coconuts

figs

grapefruits

grapes

kiwis

mangoes

nectarines

papayas

peaches

pineapples

plums

pomegranate

watermelons

all other fruits

Healthy Fats

avocados

oils (extra virgin, virgin, unrefined, cold pressed preferred): avocado oil, almond oil, butter (grass fed), coconut oil, ghee, flax oil, macadamia oil, olive oil, sesame oil, walnut oil

olives

omega-3 (from cold-water fish, flax, or chia seeds)

raw unroasted nuts and seeds and nut butters: almonds, Brazil nuts, cashews, hazelnuts, macadamia nuts, pecans, pumpkin seeds, sesame seeds, sunflower seeds

Herbs/Spices

basil

black pepper

cayenne pepper

chili pepper (capsaicin)

cilantro

cinnamon

cloves

cumin

dill

fennel

garlic

mustard seed

nutmeg

oregano

paprika

parsley

peppermint

rosemary

sage

tarragon

thyme

turmeric (curcumin)

Beverages

bone broth or vegetable broth

filtered still water

green tea

herbal teas

kombucha

organic, unsweetened
almond, cashew, hemp,
sunflower, coconut,
pumpkin seed milks

organic low-acid coffee

raw vegetable juices

sparkling water
(unsweetened and
in moderation)

"Sometimes" Foods and Treats

alcohol intake (1 to
2 servings a day, red
wine is preferred)

organic dark chocolate
(72% cacao or higher)

organic stevia

raw honey or molasses

Foods to Exclude or Reduce

Proteins: Avoid or reduce your intake of conventionally raised animal proteins, deep-fried protein sources, and processed meat products such as bologna, hot dogs, salami, and sausages.

Carbohydrates: Avoid or reduce intake of packaged, convenience noodles, processed chips, and crackers, and other processed carbohydrates (look for ingredients and fiber content), fried vegetables, and starches. Look out for excess sources of fructose found in table sugar, high-fructose corn syrup, agave syrup, and fruit juices. Limit high glycemic index foods. Keep in mind that refined grains behave like simple starches, and since they are easily digested and rapidly absorbed, the rise in blood glucose and subsequent insulin spike can cause the same inflammatory response as sugar.

Fats: Avoid or reduce your intake of processed, damaged trans fats (hydrogenated fats) like those typically found in prepared foods and margarines. Damage can also occur with fat in meats when grilled or broiled on high heat. Avoid fried foods and heat-refined oils.

Food-Preparation Methods

The way you cook and prepare your food can not only influence its nutrient density but, in some instances, actually make the food more pro-inflammatory. This process occurs when proteins and fats produce advanced glycation end products (AGEs) as a result of heat exposure. Exposure to these AGEs promote inflammation and can thus trigger heart disease, obesity, aging, and arthritis. AGEs are created when food is cooked at high temperature or grilled. In order to avoid this, opt for going slow with low temperatures like stewing, poaching, braising. If you are going to be grilling foods, marinate them.

Certain foods (beans, seeds, nuts, and grains) also come with certain recommendations for proper preparation techniques. You may be aware of some of the concerns with lectins, phytic acids, and enzyme inhibitors and/or you may have read some of the recent best-sellers on the subject. Lectins are proteins that bind to carbohydrates and cell membranes. In nature, lectins provide a line of defense to plants and that defense mechanism is what may cause problems with digestion as they resist being broken down in the gut and can stand strong in the face of an acidic environment. Their resiliency can potentially cause damage to intestinal tissue if they are eaten in large amounts or if you consume undercooked beans or grains. Phytic acids are considered to be anti-nutrients because they block the absorption of minerals such as iron, zinc, and calcium in the digestive tract and can contribute to deficiencies. Enzyme inhibitors (the name is somewhat self-explanatory) block enzymes that help break down food in the digestive process.

While we're not going to debate the pros and cons of eliminating these compounds and, ultimately, their sources in your diet, there are steps you can take to reduce them and thus reduce their potential to cause an inflammatory response. These steps include soaking, sprouting, fermenting, and cooking.

Become an expert at reading food and ingredient labels. The best-case scenario would be if your diet consisted of foods that didn't require these labels, but I am a realist. If a food label has more than five ingredients or if sugars (look for words ending in "ose") is in the first three ingredients, or if you can't pronounce the ingredients, it's most likely not going to support your goals. Just because something is organic, that does not mean it should always be considered healthy.

For example, an organic diet soda or an organic fried snack chip can be both organic and even vegan, but that doesn't make it healthy. Sometimes we lose sight of how sugar on a label translates into table sugar for a visual. Every 4 grams of sugar = 1 teaspoon of sugar. Take a look at some items you typically use and calculate what the sugar intake would look like in table sugar. (Yes, a spoonful of sugar makes the medicine go down, because it's a vicious cycle.)

Stem Cell–Supporting Lifestyle Changes

A major takeaway for your entire journey here is to look at ways to improve the quality of the air you breathe, the water you drink, and the food you eat. We covered this extensively in the previous few chapters.

Stay Active

Lack of activity destroys the good condition of every human being, while movement and methodical physical exercise save it and preserve it."

—Plato

The usual rule of thumb for health is to get at least 150 minutes of activity per week. If you're aiming to lose weight or improve health, that number goes up to 250 to 300 minutes per week. A different quote I have in my office says, "What fits your busy schedule better, exercising for one hour a day or being dead for twenty-four hours per day?"

We reviewed the evidence for exercise on aging and stem cell support. Consider ways you can become more active and incorporate movement into your daily routine. Activity doesn't have to mean becoming a gym rat. Start off small, make it fun, and involve family or friends. Begin with 10-minute spurts of movement at least two to three times per day. The key is to do something that you enjoy. Set a goal that's realistic. Maybe even make use of that wearable device you probably already own.

I look at exercise as the gift that keeps on giving, and when looking at things from an ROI framework, it's not just about the calories burned but more about the fact that movement helps you to live longer, stronger, with a better quality of life and stronger mental health and self-image. Plus, it helps with digestion, so it even helps your overall gut health.

Get Adequate Sleep

We'll go into greater detail on this in Chapter 8.

Stay Hydrated

Recall our discussion in Chapter 2 about water and its job description. Aim to drink at least half of your body weight or target body weight in ounces of fluid per day. As we look to help support our stem cells, remember "the solution to pollution is dilution." Drinking plenty of fluids helps to detoxify your organs (liver, kidneys, intestines), ensuring they have the necessary water to excrete toxins and waste products. Use the color of your urine as a guide. If it's dark, you need to drink more. Shoot to have pale-colored urine (some foods and supplements may change the color of your urine). If you feel thirsty, you're already falling way behind on maintaining adequate hydration. Drink up to your stem cells, my friends!

Reduce Stress

There's a reason why the phrase "stress kills" exists. None of us are immune from it. Stress is a fact of life, and a certain amount of stress is necessary for overall health. But our current society has many of us dealing with an overabundance of stress. This chronic exposure to stress triggers a downward spiral of a pro-inflammatory cascade in the body that can cause deleterious effects on every body system and your stem cells. While there are a multitude of interventions one can choose to help with stress reduction and countless books, blogs, apps, and podcasts, I like to use the simple and easy stress stoppers. Deep breathing is a great place to start.

My personal favorite is the 4-7-8 method. This is great not only for stress but also to prepare for sleep. When using the 4-7-8 technique, you focus on your breathing pattern. To begin, breathe in quietly through the nose for a count of 4 seconds, then hold your breath for a count of 7 seconds. Finally, exhale forcefully through the mouth, pursing the lips and making a "whoosh" sound, for a count of 8 seconds. Repeat for at least four cycles.

Finally, the best stress reliever is engaging in activities that bring you joy.

To Supplement or Not to Supplement?

Work with a knowledgeable clinician to evaluate the impact that your diet, lifestyle, medical history, and medications can have on you and to determine any need for supportive supplements. Examples include vitamin D, resveratrol, curcumin, vitamin C, quercetin, and glucosamine.

Being a realist, I think that if you are seriously going to adopt any of the fasting styles we discussed and especially if you are starting off depleted, it may be of benefit to use a good-quality multivitamin/mineral supplement with an omega-3 supplement two to three times per week. The best-case scenario would be to obtain a comprehensive micronutrient blood panel with a functional provider to assess your current status and develop a repletion plan.

Chapter 7

THE ROLE OF MICRONUTRIENT SUPPLEMENTS

You might still be questioning whether or not you want to use supplements. Remember that when you are actively fasting or calorie restricting in order to activate the power within the cell, adding supplements can work against you. But what about in between rounds of targeted dietary changes? Dietary supplements are definitely a hot topic my patients ask me about almost daily.

This discussion comes up so frequently that I even wrote an article on the subject for a recent issue of *Lancaster County Physician* magazine to help doctors better understand how to address this concern with their patients. I will share that discussion with you here as well. I will begin by saying that I do believe in the use of supportive and targeted supplementation. However, supplements are meant to be in addition to, not in place of, a healthy diet. You cannot out-supplement a bad diet. But if you were to look at the supplements in the media, you'd think we simply could not live without them.

In order to understand dietary supplements, it's worth beginning by looking at their definition, according to the Dietary Supplement Health and Education Act of 1994: A product (other than tobacco) that is intended to supplement the diet, be taken by mouth, and contains one or more dietary ingredients:

- Macronutrients

- Vitamins, minerals, amino acids

- Herbs or other botanicals

- "Other" dietary substances

Just how common is supplement use? Data from the National Health and Nutrition Examination Survey (NHANES 1999 to 2012) describes the use of dietary supplements in the United States:

- Fifty percent of adults, 70 percent of older adults, and one-third of children are consuming dietary supplements.

- The most commonly used product is a multivitamin.

- Supplement use increases with age and differs by sex, education, race/ethnicity, family income, physical activity, health insurance coverage, smoking, and prescription drug use.

- Usage may help with meeting nutrient recommendations.

- Users tend to have been previously diagnosed with chronic conditions (e.g., high cholesterol, diabetes).

- Supplements are used mainly to improve or maintain health, prevent health problems, and supplement the diet.

The data from NHANES also shows us that Americans are using dietary supplements beyond their intended use. Reasons for this can possibly include:

- the idea that taking supplements acts like an "insurance policy" of sorts
- medical self-treatment
- the idea that use provides a degree of invincibility

Although Americans have demonstrated high supplement use, there is a lack of general agreement on whether individual vitamins and minerals or their combinations should be taken as supplements for cardiovascular disease prevention or treatment. What does exist is the standard recommendation of consumption of a balanced diet as part of a healthy lifestyle. Our neighbors to the north take it one step further: The Canadian Cancer Society recommends that a supplement of 1,000 IU vitamin D be taken in fall and winter.

The Literature on the Benefits of Dietary Supplements

Nutritional research has repeatedly exhibited an inverse association between various foods and lower rates of cardiovascular disease, cancer, and other major morbidity and mortality. However, the difference between food's association with health and that of dietary supplements suggests numerous factors to consider. Is it the food matrix, one or more of its nutrients, patterns of food combinations, or the function of other confounding non-dietary factors that contribute to the synergistic effects?

The US Preventive Service Task Force conducted a 2014 review and issued:

- A recommendation against ß-carotene or vitamin E supplements for the prevention of cardiovascular disease or cancer.

- A conclusion that the current evidence is insufficient to assess the balance of benefits and harms of multivitamins for the prevention of cardiovascular disease or cancer.

- A conclusion that the current evidence is insufficient to assess the balance of benefits and harms of single- or paired-nutrient supplements (except ß-carotene and vitamin E) for the prevention of cardiovascular disease or cancer.

Additionally, a different study reported finding "generally moderate- or low-quality evidence for preventive benefits for folic acid for total cardiovascular disease, and folic acid and B vitamins for stroke; no effect for multivitamins, vitamins C, D, ß-carotene, calcium, and selenium; and increased risk with antioxidant mixtures and niacin (with a statin) for all-cause mortality.

A Closer Look at Antioxidant Supplements

As we gain a greater understanding of cellular defense mechanisms, there is a tangible shift in the literature regarding the use of antioxidants, specifically when promoting their use to support cellular defense. We've spent a lot of time looking at specific tools we can use to optimize stem cells, and during times where we want to trigger autophagy, antioxidant symptoms would work against us. They could provide a crutch for cells to hang on when we really are trying to hasten their demise. In order to maintain overall cellular health and wellness, oxidation processes must be in balance; the body is always seeking to maintain homeostasis.

Numerous factors, such as intense exercise, emotional stress, depressed mood, poor diet, and micronutrient deficiencies all serve as stressors to the body, increasing production of reactive oxygen species (ROS). However, that does not mean that all sources of increased ROS production are inherently bad. While the research strongly supports that increased free radical formation is usually a result of tissue damage by a disease or toxin, in some circumstances ROS may be employing a protective role, such as helping to down-regulate inflammation. Exercise has been shown to have an overall anti-inflammatory effect, despite its acute production of ROS. In fact, one study showed how the use of antioxidant supplementation had a negative impact on exercise by blocking the positive effects exercise has on metabolism.[9]

While it is tempting to think that when it comes to antioxidant supplementation, "an ounce of prevention is worth a pound of cure," this is certainly not the case. Antioxidant supplements do not offer the same health benefits as antioxidants in foods. In fact, high-dose antioxidant supplements generally do no good and may cause harm. Clinical studies call our attention to the lack of evidence supporting a benefit from high consumption of nutritional antioxidants for protection against disease in persons without deficiencies.

For disease prevention, the evidence is more in favor of consumption versus supplementation. The key to the usefulness of antioxidants may be in the synergy of their naturally occurring form, alongside the importance of lifestyle interventions. It is also important to note that antioxidant supplements can act as pro-oxidants and actually become oxidative stress inducers

---

9 Ristow, Zarse, Oberbach et al., "Antioxidants Prevent Health-Promoting Effects of Physical Exercise in Humans," 8665–70.

when taken at levels significantly above the recommended dietary intakes.

When Should I Consider a Dietary Supplement?

With a lack of strong evidence supporting the advantages of supplements, we must weigh the possible benefits against the risks when considering their use. Because supplement users are more likely to be female, older, physically active adults who consume a healthier diet, usage may be a marker for a healthy lifestyle. Therefore, an irony exists: The most common users are often the ones who need supplements the least. Furthermore, it's important to remember that supplement labels fail to note if they exceed the recommended upper limit (UL) of a nutrient. American adults do not exceed the ULs from foods alone, only with supplements.

Individuals who should seek guidance to determine the need for targeted, short-term, supportive supplementation include:

- Those with poor nutrient intakes from food

- Those consuming low-calorie diets

- Those avoiding specific groups of foods (e.g., vegans)

- Those with medical conditions that impair digestion, absorption, or use of nutrients

- Older adults, who may benefit from B12

What to Look for in a Supplement

The FDA does not approve supplements nor register them. While good manufacturing practices (GMPs) are required, they are set by the manufacturer and do not set contamination limits, ingredient identity parameters, or testing methods. In fact, 54 percent of GMP inspections in FY 2018 resulted in citations of infractions, most commonly for identification of ingredient issues. Common problems with supplements include:

- Too little or no ingredient

- Too much ingredient

- Inadequate labeling to describe ingredients

- Poor-quality ingredients

- Spoilage of oils

- Contamination with heavy metals

- Inadequate disintegration of pills

- Unapproved label claims

In choosing supplements, stick with reputable brands that have been evaluated by third-party labs for safety, authenticity, and effectiveness. Be cautious with products that have "proprietary blends." Consider using ConsumerLab.com (nominal annual subscription required) for up-to-date product reviews, testing, and quality certifications.

Key Points

There are a few key points to consider when evaluating your potential micronutrient status. Have you had micronutrient testing, and do your labs illustrate the presence or absence of micronutrient deficiencies or other metabolic barriers? What, if any, genomic information is available? What nutrient depletions may be occurring as a result of medication use?

The current common theme of personalizing of nutritional choices pertains in this area, too, as there may be some instances where micronutrients, particularly antioxidant support through supplementation, may be needed. Therefore, the choice of the correct form, dose, standardization, product, and timing of a supplement is paramount. However, based on the current body of evidence, these more simplistic recommendations are in order:

- Consume a diet that naturally provides antioxidants, one that is nutrient-dense but not calorically dense.

- Increase consumption of brightly colored fruits, vegetables, and whole grains.

- Focus on supporting an antioxidant lifestyle—get plenty of exercise. Exercise will help to give your cells an edge to better detoxify a large quantity of ROS, thereby reducing the negative effects caused by free radicals.

- Refrain from tobacco use, limit alcohol, reduce stress, get proper rest, and avoid processed and poor-quality foods.

Chapter 8

BIOHACKING

Now here is a new and interesting emerging topic. The title *bio-hacking* alone may sound a little frightening and intimidating. Or it may have you thinking, "Here we go again with sci-fi references." Biohacking is also known as "DIY biology." It really is not as intimidating as it sounds, nor are we talking about doing anything illicit or illegal. Though the term "hacking" tends to stir up thoughts of breaking into something—emails, bank accounts, or computer systems—that's not what we're talking about here. Biohacking is all about improving your biology through lifestyle changes, which is a perfect add-on philosophy to activating and optimizing our stem cells. Biohackers do this through a combination of nutritional, medical, and even electronic tools.

Biohackers aim to exert some degree of control over their environment, sleep, nutrition, fitness, and brain. Data is very important and useful to the biohacker, so wearable devices and tracking apps are pretty commonplace.

Young blood transfusions and fecal transplants are examples of some extreme hacks, but biohacking doesn't have to be hard or even require a major overhaul to your routine. Many biohackers use small gradual changes that can make some pretty significant improvements to one's mind and body, thereby producing significant life-changing effects. What are some of these hacks that we can do to improve our biology?

Biohacking Your Environment

Light Therapy

For starters, you can look at the amount of light that your body and brain are being exposed to on a daily basis. Infrared light therapy is a common intervention for biohackers. Light exposure is needed to help our bodies in our brain to function at their peak capabilities. We won't even get into the debate surrounding the true prevalence of Americans walking around with suboptimal levels of vitamin D. But if you haven't had yours checked, it's a pretty good idea to do so. A word to the wise: While many lab tests show normal ranges of 30 to 100 ng/mL, the optimal range is generally considered to be from 50 to 80 ng/mL (ng/mL stands for nanograms per milliliter).

In today's rat-race society, how often are you actually spending enough time outdoors to get natural light therapy and a dose of vitamin D directly from the sun? Light and vitamin D provide benefits from a physiological as well as a psychological standpoint. In fact, if you're dealing with depression-like symptoms and you haven't had your vitamin D level checked, that's another valid reason to do so. Given the barriers that exist to obtaining adequate sunlight, research has shown that our bodies respond well to red and near-infrared light wavelengths ranging from 600 to 900 nanometers (nm). The light is absorbed and activates a series of metabolic and nervous system processes.

For biohackers, red light therapy has become a popular tool as it also helps relieve pain, reduce inflammation, and restore optimal function. Because it's a noninvasive intervention, it may be an easy add-on to your daily wellness routine. Red light therapy is touted as improving skin tone and producing anti-aging effects on the skin, and enhancing muscle recovery.

Additional ways to biohack your environment include: saunas, cryotherapy chambers, salt rooms, float tanks, and more simple changes, such as adding salt lamps and targeted placement of plants, or just taking a good old cold shower or ice bath.

Biohacking Your Nutrition

Intermittent Fasting

Intermittent fasting (IF) falls into this biohacking category and we've already spent a significant amount of time highlighting all of the benefits that fasting provides.

Elimination Diets

Many biohackers are proponents of using elimination diets to determine if they have any food sensitivities or food intolerances such as histamines. Then using the information they learn through their elimination diet program, they alter their food choices accordingly.

Nutrigenomics

Nutrigenomics is the science behind how the food we eat interacts with our genes. From a biohacking standpoint, if you have had genetic testing done you can tailor and optimize the nutrient composition of your diet and supplement regimen based on your nutrigenomic results.

Blood Tests

Even your routine blood testing can be viewed as biohacking if you actually take the information and use it to make targeted changes. The sky's the limit here, especially for those with the financial means to run more in-depth blood, saliva, stool, and hair tests in order to target as many areas as possible where changes could be made.

Biohacking Your Sleep

Sleep can seem like a rare commodity for many of us, and sleep deprivation, including a lack of quality sleep, is a common barrier to optimal health and wellness. Wearable devices that can track your sleep are common tools for biohackers. When trying to "hack" your sleep, some rules of thumb are:

- Support your natural circadian rhythm through exposure to light and darkness.

- Get some exercise, but not too late in the day.

- Watch your diet: Try not to eat or drink anything (except water) for three hours before bed.

- Cut off caffeine by 2 p.m., or noon if you struggle with sleep issues.

- Avoid exposing yourself to anything that may drive nighttime tension or anxiety.

- Develop a nighttime-bedtime routine: Set a sleep and wake schedule and stick with it, even on the weekends.

Biohacking Your Muscle and Bone Structure

Bone Density

Following along the same lines as tools aimed at reducing inflammation and joint pain, another area of focus for biohacking is our bone health and bone density. Biohackers will utilize any number of interventions. These can include stem cell or PRP injections, supplements, and even certain exercise machines focused on "skeletal strength conditioning."

Muscle Hacking

Changes in this category that biohackers use include saunas, as well as other techniques, such as occlusion training and oxygen-restriction training. Occlusion training uses an elastic band wrapped around the muscle you are targeting during your workout. It is intended to work like tourniquet; proponents claim it stimulates growth hormone release and muscle growth, and improves strength training.

Oxygen restriction training requires the use of an oxygen-restriction mask, also known as an altitude-training masks. The hack here is, by restricting the amount of oxygen you have access to on each breath, you trigger your body to move more hemoglobin, the oxygen-carrying component of your red blood cells, to your muscles. This is also thought to improve your body's ability to adapt to hormonal and immune system responses.

Biohacking Your Brain

Items in this category include meditation, inversion therapy, electrical brain stimulation, neurofeedback, light therapy, brain games, brainwave entrainment, and over-the-counter supplements such as omega-3, DHA, magnesium, vitamin D, turmeric, the B vitamins, choline, and glutathione. A subcategory of smart drugs and cognitive enhancers, supplements, and other substances called nootropics are also favorites among biohackers due to their benefits on cognitive function. These can include caffeine, low-dose lithium, modafinil, forskolin, L-theanine, bacopa monnieri, and piracetam. Illegal psychedelic substances such as microdoses of LSD and psilocybin (magic mushrooms) are also used by some biohackers to help improve cognitive function.

If you are considering biohacking for yourself, you'll see that anything that provides you with information on how your body is functioning provides a greater opportunity for you to identify ways to optimize those mechanical functions. There is a subgroup of biohackers called Grinders who take it one step further with devices and actually implant computer chips in their bodies. (Here we go back to science fiction: I start thinking of cyborgs when I think about some of the extremes people are going to.)

Overall, some forms of biohacking have merit and are relatively easy to implement. They are also easy to quit if you do not see a benefit or if there is a side effect. Other forms of biohacking, however, require much more time, as well as a financial investment and other interventions that can be pretty risky or illegal.

Do your own research and decide for yourself what types of biohacking interventions you want to make part of your routine. I also encourage you to speak with a knowledgeable licensed clinician who is an expert on the hacks that you are considering before you try anything on your own. Remember, there is a significant difference between someone who is an expert in an area and someone who is a social media influencer. When it comes to topics regarding health and wellness, there are far more influencers than experts out there, so be judicious with your sources of expert information and advice.

Chapter 9

DISCUSSIONS WITH THE EXPERTS

During the course of conducting research for this book, I had the remarkable opportunity to interview a few of the top experts in the field of fasting, fasting-mimicking diets, and stem cell clinical research. Much of their research has been cited in the notes section if you choose to read further on the scientific research.

Key Points from My Discussion with Dr. Sebastian Brandhorst

Sebastian Brandhorst, PhD, has scientific training based on a vast background in cell biology, molecular biology, medicine, and biochemistry, all of which are highly relevant to his focus on biogerontology research to identify the mechanisms underlying cellular protection, as well as health and lifespan-regulation, and their translation into clinical applications. Dr. Brandhorst has performed research related to aging in yeast and *C. elegans* since 2009, after which he began to utilize mouse models to study the role of growth hormone/insulin-like growth factor 1

(IGF-1) signaling as a major regulatory pathway that modulates lifespan and age-associated diseases/pathologies—particularly cancer. Subsequently, he focused on the role and application of short-term starvation, low-calorie and/or low-protein diets, and fasting-mimicking diets on health and lifespan in preclinical to clinical studies.

It seems like biohacking has become quite a buzz word in the blogging world. You've published many articles on fasting and fasting-mimicking diets. The article that you just published in March looks at inflammatory bowel disease and the impact it had on the intestinal stem cells—Can elaborate on that?

My angle on this is usually more on the diet side of things. I think the one advantage that you have is you use a diet. I think the diet is almost causing the entire organism to change its metabolism. And with that, you have very cell-specific effects; for example, changes in how stem cells behave or whether it is an upregulation in stress response, or changes in the muscle with regard to insulin sensitivity.

All that is induced by just a single intervention. I think that's the big advantage with regard to the diet, obviously. Yes, it was a low-calorie intervention and that forces cells to identify mechanisms to sort of optimize their metabolism. That can be obviously using autophagy, or changing in the way they metabolize fatty acids and so on. So for stem cells, I think that the important thing is and what we see is that you need to have a period of low calories where you induce autophagy so you lose cells.

The prime example in our study was that the liver shrank during four days on fasting in a mouse, which obviously has a high metabolism. But it's just by using the fasting-mimicking diet or fasting that the liver really shrinks quite dramatically from before like 30 to 40 percent. And within just a couple of days of just refeeding, all this gets sort of reestablished, indicating that there's really a dramatic turnover of losing cells. Hopefully these are all the damaged cells that can't respond to the signal.

At the same time, once you provide food again, the whole system re-expands. I think that's really where stem cells in all organs become really prominent and play a prominent role. You have the induction of stem cells in the liver. We show it in the gut. Interestingly, we also show an induction of neogenesis, which is in the brain, obviously doesn't really lose mass. It doesn't sound like cells die off rapidly. We still see an induction there. It is really a systemic effect on many of the stem cells, specialized cells in the muscle. Lots going on.

One of the questions that I often get from patients who are interested in fasting involves comparing the fasting-mimicking diet to University of Southern California's or yours and Doctor Longo's fasting-mimicking plan, which is definitely lower in protein and higher in carbohydrates, because it is totally plant based.

How do you answer the opposite side of the fence: the folks who are doing ketogenic, fasting-mimicking plans where they're doing much higher-fat, higher-protein, lower-carb? Have you seen any comparisons with that? Does that side of the coin see as much stem cell activation or optimization of stem cells as the FMD plan?

Our FMD diet is technically a fat-rich diet. It's a little protein, moderate amount of the complex carbs, and then relatively high fat. It's not as high as the ketogenic diet. Obviously, if you consider the definition of ketogenic diet with very high fat, protein with a very minimal amount of carb, the reason why we don't do this is, generally speaking, high-protein diets or diets rich in protein, are usually the ones identified as being the worst outcome for lifespan and health. So why? Well, you can have short-term effects such as weight loss, which is the great motivator for a lot of people.

These diets are usually not the ones that are being generally associated with longevity in epidemiological studies in mouse studies, monkey studies. So that's why we're staying away from it. And reality is we haven't really done it. We have done a comparison for multiple sclerosis, where we compared a ketogenic diet or one round of the fasting-mimicking diet, followed by a Mediterranean diet. And in that case, I think especially the quality of life for all those subjects with MS was actually improved in people with FMD and the Mediterranean diet, more so than in the ketogenic diet. So we think FMD is better.

We're really not doing comprehensive studies. The real reasons why are it is almost cost prohibitive. They're usually very long studies. It's hard for us to compare everything. We're trying to do this now in a very complex matter and in a large animal study that was planning to start in like October or November. But it's we are essentially making baby steps at this point.

In terms of optimizing stem cells. Have you had any experience with looking at how genetics factor into it? When we look at the expanding fields of nutrigenetics, epigenetics, and nutrigenomics, can you comment on this in terms of stem cell activation?

The short answer, no. And to expand on that, we're doing a little bit of RNA study right now and we're actually working on getting some metabolomics done with a group in Italy right now. Nothing is officially analyzed. I'm still sort of collecting samples to be sent out.

The only omics I can probably comment on was based on the inflammatory bowel disease paper where obviously you can sort of see changes in the microbiome following a diet and that sort of has systemic changes on regeneration, rejuvenation, and sort of like the immune system. That's probably the most extensive one we have done so far.

Have you had anybody raise objections to the constituents of the fasting-mimicking plan—for example, those who might be supporters of Dr. Gundry and the whole plant paradox (lectins, phytates, things like that). When you look at the ingredients in ProLon, have people pushed back because of that? Do you get any comments on that?

Sure. It's very hard to customize diets individually to every person and every intolerance. You know, do they want to eat nightshades or nuts? "And I don't like olives. I don't like that soup," so reality, if we can, on our end we're trying to accommodate everybody. But this is sort of what we have is what we can work with right now. And I think there are probably ways to sort of begin to customize things a little bit more. But on my end, I think we're doing the clinical trials as essentially a proof of concept that it works and there's a learning curve for everyone in there. It doesn't mean that we all disagree with *Plant Paradox* or all the other publications that are out there on various diets and all that. But, you know, it's really just a matter of life for us—it's cost prohibitive.

If you had to list three or four top foods to activate or optimize stem cells, based on your research, what would you include?

Tough question. Really tough question. It isn't just specific ingredients. I think that's what I'm struggling with right now. I think it is a systemic effect that you get by the combination of in this case, the diet. And I think it goes to a point that I generally like to make. It's like we're consuming foods, we're not consuming food on an individual level. We're not just saying let's just eat leucine and then everything goes bad or, let's eat phytoestrogens and everything goes good or so. With dietary interventions there are a lot of things that go hand in hand.

I don't think we understand everything that happens right now. I don't think I actually can point out two or three components where we feel like this is probably what happened. I think low protein probably plays a role to get to the point where reducing glucose and IGF-1, I think we've shown before the moment you reverse that, you lose most of the effect. All of this linked to carbs, metabolism, protein. I don't think I have a good answer for you.

In terms of research on stem cells, looking at fasting and circadian rhythms, do you have an opinion—if you're going to be using fasting and fasting-mimicking diets—is it best for the fast to coincide with a circadian rhythm?

Yeah, I actually do think that's the major benefit of this. And I think, when you go back to looking at a lot of the work that has been done on caloric restriction, also in animals for the longest time, it has been ignored. But actually when you feed the mice, they're hungry, they eat everything, and then they fast for the next 20 hours or so, I think that has been traditionally overlooked as a component of caloric restriction. I think that's why I actually think time-restricted feeding is for the great majority of people, actually, a fairly easy-to-do application that has, and will have, if done right, a lot of health benefits.

I do think that the benefit of the fasting-mimicking diet now is obviously also people tend to not overeat late at night. With the

FMD you are calorically restricted. But also the way you consume food is changing that pattern of life. Do you wake up early? Have your coffee, go to work, snack the entire day, come home late and then, you know, by 9:00, 9:30, have your largest meal of the day thirty minutes before you go to bed? I absolutely believe that there is a benefit of the FMD. I believe it forces people to time respect their food intake.

I think that's where you get a lot of benefits from, because now you're lining up your food intake to when your metabolic hormones actually work, which is, they go up in the morning and then it's sort of like everything shuts down when it gets dark. So, yes, absolutely. I do think it plays a big role.

Say you had somebody ask, "What's the easiest thing I can do on my own to improve my stem cells?" Would the FMD be the number one intervention?

Yes. But I'm totally biased. I do think that what we've seen so far is that the FMD is a great tool. That is excluding comments on cost or obviously, you pay for a convenience buying the product. But there's a lot of research that went into what L-Nutra's providing and obviously you pay for what you get more. I think it has great application for people because it's not a major lifestyle intervention.

It's not always easy to break habits that you established over the last 20, 30, 40, 50, 60 years. And everything we've seen so far really seems to be beneficial, particularly when you look at it and say, look, this actually seems to be working the best for people that really need an intervention. If you are already healthy, you probably don't need to do it that often, but you can use it as an intervention to sort of bring you back on track. Everybody I talked to, unless they are very lean to begin with, feel like it's that easy to follow interventions five days. Totally doable. I think that. It's easy to make that recommendation to people.

Do you have any advice on stem cell activation in the use of dietary manipulation that you'd want to share?

There is no secret, obviously. Whatever we have done, this is published. So luckily the data is available. I always caution when translating mouse work into humans. But so far as we know, we've seen that the diet is at least safe and feasible for the great majority of people. We are hopeful that we can continue to really use the diet in multiple different diseases to self-expand, because it's always the question, we all talk about the use of the FMD and diabetes. I think we're getting better and better. We have more trials. We're close to 25 trials planned or ongoing. We'll have more data coming up in the next year.

Key Points from My Discussion with Dr. Stephen Anton

Dr. Stephen Anton is an associate professor and chief of clinical research within the Department of Aging and Geriatric Research at the University of Florida. His specific research interests are in the role that lifestyle factors and natural compounds play in influencing obesity, cardiovascular disease, and metabolic disease conditions during aging.

Over the past fifteen years, he has successfully obtained multiple grants and conducted several clinical trials examining the effects that lifestyle-based interventions have on biological and functional outcomes relevant to metabolic disease and aging. With more than 130 peer-reviewed scientific articles and book chapters, his research has been recognized both nationally as well as internationally. In 2017, Dr. Anton was awarded a UF Term Professorship, a distinction given to top professors at the University of Florida.

I'd like to discuss with you the research that you've done on the fasting side, not necessarily from the perspective of stem cell activation, but in terms of the general benefits that fasting provides as an intervention.

There was such a study that showed lifespan was extended by about 11 percent by simply restricting the time to calories. The general idea, although we still need more clear data, is that the longer you fast, the greater the increase in stem cell regeneration/number available to help when the fast is over to help repair.

One of the questions that I have in terms of fasting in stem cell activation is, where's the fine line between activating a significant amount of autophagy? At what point do you cross that line? When might fasting actually work against you?

Yes. These are the questions, these are great questions that I get often but I have maybe somewhat good news. We did a human clinical trial with medical students that looked at the effect of intermittent fasting on markers of autophagy and mitochondria. We published it not too long ago. At the time I'm sure we've reviewed the literature and at least as a human trial that shows the gene expression of CERT3 was significantly increased following the fasting protocol.

The other autophagy-related genes were that maybe there was one or two that also were elevated. But at least it shows in human clinical model even in basically younger, healthier people that there was this uptick in markers of autophagy and cell repair. So that's one human trial that I just remember that we were part of. But then your other question. I mean it's a great question, and really hard to have great, clear, easy answers to that. But I would say the best one diet is the one that people will consistently do, because if they won't do it, then it doesn't really ultimately matter. 24 hours or 5:2, versus 16:8. So if they won't do it, then it doesn't really matter.

In your experience and in your research, have you seen any difference between fasting and prolonged water fasting?

That is what many people seem to have these great benefits from in terms of rebuilding the immune system. Reactivating mitochondria and autophagy and all of the benefits that we think are possible seem to occur from the longer water fast. I haven't dug into your question more directly, though I haven't seen any clinical comparison of a fasting-mimicking diet. I know that they said that there is this concern about the microbiome or other potential factors, related to immunity, maybe.

But I don't know of any human study that would support that happening. These are the questions I'm asking myself, too, because why? What is the optimal, "best prescription"? I do think the literature that I reviewed and I've presented shows that the time-restricted feeding approach seems to be a little bit better at maintaining lean mass than maybe longer fasting period approaches. But that could be because people simply just don't eat enough during the time period when they are eating to compensate for the amount of energy they burn while they were fasting.

And that was one of the reported challenges in our human clinical trial, that there was an every-other-day feeding where they reported difficulty actually eating enough calories on the day when they were allowed to basically feed. I do think there are a lot of options to consider and they're all probably beneficial in one way or the other, especially compared to not fasting. In my view, it would be if you start with the time-restricted feeding and people start to adapt to that. Start to think about the longer-term fast and experiment a little bit with the 24 hour and if that's okay, go a little longer because it does seem that the benefits are increased with longer periods.

How often should you use fasting as an intervention? And then how do you make sure within your fasting window that, when you are eating, you're still meeting your micronutrient needs?

I would say related to the micronutrients is if they were theoretically getting sufficient micronutrients with their previous diet, that's the first question. That's a big question. But presuming they were then, they theoretically should if they still eat the same food, and just the same quantity, just in a shorter time period. That shouldn't change.

Maybe the point would be, how important it is to tell people just because you fast doesn't give you a license to eat crappy food when you do eat, because then you're losing the nutrients. My point is theoretically it should still be there, but maybe it's just simply not eating as often reduces the likelihood. That is a potential concern.

It's especially concerning in the people who are doing the one-meal-a-day-type of fast. How are you physically going to be able to consume the necessary amount of servings of even produce in that one meal, to really make sure you're covering your needs?

I thought about the one meal a day a couple of times and on the surface it's great idea because you can fast for so long. But on the other hand, I just think it's really hard to just get the calories you need in that single meal. Maybe not that hard for the calories, but certainly the micronutrients. But at least personally,

I find it not the most energizing way to live. Some people maybe do great on it. But for me, usually I need about two meals a day. Sometimes a snack.

Do you feel strongly, though, that if you're going to be using intermittent fasting, the greatest benefit is if you're eating within your circadian rhythm? There are proponents who strongly believe that if you're going to be fasting, your windows should be from 7 a.m. to 3 p.m., or 8 a.m. to 4 p.m., making sure you have breakfast rather than eating later in the day.

I think it's more about what works best for the person. I do think it's good not to eat a huge meal at night, though. Having said all that, I sleep better when I have less food in my stomach.

That's balancing the optimal versus the realistic.

Yes, exactly!

FINAL THOUGHTS

In order to chart a course, one needs a point of origin. One of my main themes in my daily work is *enlighten, energize, and empower* those with whom I have contact with. This theme has also guided me in writing this book. By enlightening readers, I help to facilitate your understanding on a health concern by explaining it or by bringing new information or facts to your attention. By energizing readers, I assist your ability to make some active changes and how to make you feel energetic or eager for the steps toward your optimal wellness. By empowering readers, I hope to encourage and support your ability to do something for your wellness. I hope you feel enlightened, energized, and empowered to make changes that will activate your stem cells and begin your journey toward optimizing your health and wellness. Do something today that your future self with be grateful for!

I hope that you will connect with me and share your experiences on how this book has *enlightened*, *energized*, and *empowered*. You can reach out and even work with me at www.fusionihw.com or the support site for this book, www.stemcellactivationdiet .com. Stay in touch to receive updates on additional support materials to help you on this journey or to take your wellness to the next level.

One final note, a new, revamped version of *The Biggest Loser* dubuted in January 2020. I sincerely hope this new version has learned from its past failures and that this generation of contestants will not suffer the same metabolic consequences as the former contestants have.

Cheers to you and your elevated level of health and wellness,

—Dana

BIBLIOGRAPHY

Andia, Isabel, Eva Rubio-Azpeitia, Jose Martin, and Michele Abate. "Current Concepts and Translational Uses of Platelet Rich Plasma Biotechnology," 2015. doi:10.5772/59954.

Anton, Stephen D., Azumi Hida, Kacey Heekin, Kristen Sowalsky, Christy Karabetian, Heather Mutchie, Christiaan Leeuwenburgh, Todd M. Manini, and Tracey E. Barnett. "Effects of Popular Diets without Specific Calorie Targets on Weight Loss Outcomes: Systematic Review of Findings from Clinical Trials," *Nutrients* 9, no. 8 (July 2017). doi:10.3390/nu9080822.

Anton, Stephen D., Keelin Moehl, William T. Donahoo, Krisztina Marosi, Stephanie A. Lee, Arch G. Mainous, Christiaan Leeuwenburgh, and Mark P. Mattson. "Flipping the Metabolic Switch: Understanding and Applying the Health Benefits of Fasting," *Obesity* (2018). doi:10.1002/oby.22065.

Berg, J. M., J. L. Tymoczko, and L. Stryer. "Food Intake and Starvation Induce Metabolic Changes," in *Biochemistry*, 5th Edition. New York: W. H. Freeman, 2002, www.ncbi.nlm.nih.gov/books/NBK22414.

Bindu, A. B. Hima, and B. Srilatha. "Potency of Various Types of Stem Cells and Their Transplantation," *Journal of Stem Cell Research and Therapy* 1, no. 03 (2012): 1–6. doi:10.4172/2157-7633.1000115.

Bouayed, Jaouad, and Torsten Bohn. "Exogenous Antioxidants—Double-Edged Swords in Cellular Redox State: Health Beneficial Effects at Physiologic Doses versus Deleterious Effects at High Doses," *Oxidative Medicine and Cellular Longevity* 3, no. 4 (2010): 228–37. doi:10.4161/oxim.3.4.12858.

Brandhorst, Sebastian, In Young Choi, Min Wei, Chia Wei Cheng, Sargis Sedrakyan, Gerardo Navarrete, Louis Dubeau, et al. "A Periodic Diet That Mimics Fasting Promotes Multi-System Regeneration, Enhanced Cognitive Performance, and Healthspan," *Cell Metabolism* 22, no. 1 (July 2015): 86–99. doi:10.1016/j.cmet.2015.05.012.

Cabo, Rafael De, Didac Carmona-Gutierrez, Michel Bernier, Michael N. Hall, and Frank Madeo. "Review the Search for Antiaging Interventions: From Elixirs to Fasting Regimens," *Cell* 157, no. 7 (2014): 1515–26. doi:10.1016/j.cell.2014.05.031.

Canadian Cancer Society. "Should I Take a Vitamin D Supplement?" accessed June 10, 2019, http://www.cancer.ca/en/prevention-and-screening/reduce-cancer-risk/make-healthy-choices/eat-well/should-itake-a-vitamin-d-supplement/?region.on.

Cheng, Chia-Wei, Moshe Biton, Adam L. Haber, Nuray Gunduz, George Eng, Liam T. Gaynor, Surya Tripathi, et al. "Ketone Body Signaling Mediates Intestinal Stem Cell Homeostasis and Adaptation to Diet," *Cell* 178, no. 5 (2019): 1115–1131.e15. doi:10.1016/j.cell.2019.07.048.

Cheng, Chia-Wei, Valentina Villani, Roberta Buono, Min Wei, Sanjeev Kumar, Omer H Yilmaz, Pinchas Cohen, Julie B. Sneddon, Laura Perin, and Valter D. Longo. "Fasting-Mimicking Diet Promotes Ngn3-Driven Beta-Cell Regeneration to Reverse Diabetes," *Cell* 168, no. 5 (February 2017): 775–788.e12. doi:10.1016/j.cell.2017.01.040.

Choi, In Young, Changhan Lee, and Valter D. Longo. "Nutrition and Fasting Mimicking Diets in the Prevention and Treatment of Autoimmune Diseases and Immunosenescence," *Molecular and*

Cellular Endocrinology 455 (November 5 2017): 4–12. doi:10.1016/j.mce.2017.01.042.

Cole, Brian J., Shane T. Seroyer, Giuseppe Filardo, Sarvottam Bajaj, and Lisa A. Fortier. "Platelet-Rich Plasma: Where Are We Now and Where Are We Going?" *Sports Health* 2, no. 3 (2010): 203–10. doi:10.1177/1941738110366385.

Davis, Carole, and Etta Saltos. "Dietary Recommendations and How They Have Changed over Time," *Agriculture Information Bulletin 750* (1999) 33–50. https://www.ers.usda.gov/webdocs/publications/42215/5831_aib750b_1_.pdf.

Efeyan, Alejo, William Comb, and David Sabatini, "Nutrient Sensing Mechanisms and Pathways," *Nature* 517 (January 15, 2015): 302–10. doi:10.1038/nature14190.

Fine, Eugene J., and Richard D. Feinman. "Thermodynamics of Weight Loss Diets," *Nutrition and Metabolism* 1, no. 1 (2004): 15. doi:10.1186/1743-7075-1-15.

Fothergill, Erin, Juen Guo, Lilian Howard, Jennifer C. Kerns, Nicolas D. Knuth, Robert Brychta, Kong Y. Chen, et al. "Persistent Metabolic Adaptation 6 Years After 'The Biggest Loser' Competition," *Obesity* 24, no. 8 (August 1, 2016): 1612–19. doi:10.1002/oby.21538.

Gaby, Alan. *Nutritional Medicine,* second edition. Concord, NH: Fritz Perlberg Publishing, 2017.

Gutteridge, John M. C., and Barry Halliwell. "Antioxidants: Molecules, Medicines, and Myths," *Biochemical and Biophysical Research Communications* 393, no. 4 (March 2010): 561–564. doi:10.1016/j.bbrc.2010.02.071.

Halliwell, Barry. "The Antioxidant Paradox: Less Paradoxical Now?" *British Journal of Clinical Pharmacology* 75, no. 3 (March 2013): 637–44. doi:10.1111/j.1365-2125.2012.04272.x.

Hatori, Megumi, Christopher Vollmers, Amir Zarrinpar, Luciano DiTacchio, Eric A. Bushong, Shubhroz Gill, Mathias Leblanc, et al.

"Time-Restricted Feeding without Reducing Caloric Intake Prevents Metabolic Diseases in Mice Fed a High-Fat Diet," *Cell Metabolism* 15, no. 6 (June 2012): 848–60. doi:10.1016/j.cmet.2012.04.019.

Health Resources and Services Administration, "Organ Donation Statistics," last accessed August 6, 2019, https://www.organdonor.gov/statistics-stories/statistics.html.

Jenkins, David J. A., J. David Spence, Edward L. Giovannucci, Young-In Kim, Robert Josse, Reinhold Vieth, Sonia Blanco Mejia, et al. "Supplemental Vitamins and Minerals for CVD Prevention and Treatment," *Journal of the American College of Cardiology* 71, no. 22 (June 2018): 2570–84. doi:10.1016/j.jacc.2018.04.020.

Jones, David S. *Textbook of Functional Medicine*. Gig Harbor, WA: Institute for Functional Medicine, 2010.

Lee, Jienny, Moon Sam Shin, Mi Ok Kim, Sunghee Jang, Sae Woong Oh, Mingyeong Kang, Kwangseon Jung, Yong Seek Park, and Jongsung Lee. "Apple Ethanol Extract Promotes Proliferation of Human Adult Stem Cells, Which Involves the Regenerative Potential of Stem Cells," *Nutrition Research* (2016). doi:10.1016/j.nutres.2016.06.010.

Lipski, Elizabeth. *Digestive Wellness: Strengthen the Immune System and Prevent Disease through Healthy Digestion*. New York: McGraw-Hill, 2011.

Lo, Bernard, and Lindsay Parham. "Ethical Issues in Stem Cell Research," *Endocrine Reviews* 30, no. 3 (2009): 204–13. doi:10.1210/er.2008-0031.

Longo, Valter D., and Mark P. Mattson. "Fasting: Molecular Mechanisms and Clinical Applications," *Cell Metabolism* 19, no. 2 (February 2014): 181–92. doi:10.1016/j.cmet.2013.12.008.

Mana, Miyeko D., Elaine Yih-Shuen Kuo, and Ömer H Yilmaz. "Dietary Regulation of Adult Stem Cells," *Current Stem Cell Reports* 3, no. 1 (2017): 1–8. doi:10.1007/s40778-017-0072-x.

Mihaylova, Maria M., David M. Sabatini, and Ömer H. Yilmaz. "Dietary and Metabolic Control of Stem Cell Function in Physiology and Cancer," *Cell Stem Cell* 14, no. 3 (2014): 292–305. https://doi.org/10.1016/j.stem.2014.02.008.

Mullin, Gerard E. *Integrative Gastroenterology*. New York: Oxford University Press, 2011.

Myles, Ian A. "Fast Food Fever: Reviewing the Impacts of the Western Diet on Immunity," *Nutrition Journal* 13, no. 1 (2014): 61. doi:10.1186/1475-2891-13-61.

National Institute of Health Fact Sheets, "Regenerative Medicine," last accessed August 6, 2019, https://report.nih.gov/nihfactsheets/viewfactsheet.aspx?csid=62.

National Institute of Health Stem Cell Information Home Page, last accessed August 6, 2019, https://stemcells.nih.gov/info/basics/6.htm.

Petersen, Anne Marie W, and Bente Klarlund Pedersen. "The Anti-Inflammatory Effect of Exercise," *Journal of Applied Physiology* 98, no. 4 (April 1, 2005): 1154–62. doi:10.1152/japplphysiol.00164.2004.

Pham-Huy, Lien Ai, Hua He, and Chuong Pham-Huy. "Free Radicals, Antioxidants in Disease and Health," *International Journal of Biomedical Science* 4, no. 2 (June 2008): 89–96. https://www.ncbi.nlm.nih.gov/pubmed/23675073.

Rakel, David. *Integrative Medicine*. Philadelphia, PA: Elsevier, 2017.

Ramaswamy Reddy, Shwetha Hulimavu, Roopa Reddy, N. Chaitanya Babu, and G. N. Ashok. "Stem-Cell Therapy and Platelet-Rich Plasma in Regenerative Medicines: A Review on Pros and Cons of the Technologies," *Journal of Oral and Maxillofacial Pathology* 22, no. 3 (2018): 367–74. doi:10.4103/jomfp.JOMFP_93_18.

Ristow, Michael, Kim Zarse, Andreas Oberbach, Nora Klöting, Marc Birringer, Michael Kiehntopf, Michael Stumvoll, C. Ronald Kahn, and Matthias Blüher. "Antioxidants Prevent Health-Promoting Effects of

Physical Exercise in Humans," *Proceedings of the National Academy of Sciences of the United States of America* 106, no. 21 (May 26, 2009): 8665–70. doi:10.1073/pnas.0903485106.

Shan, Zhilei, Colin D. Rehm, Gail Rogers, Mengyuan Ruan, Dong D. Wang, Frank B. Hu, Dariush Mozaffarian, Fang Fang Zhang, and Shilpa N. Bhupathiraju. "Trends in Dietary Carbohydrate, Protein, and Fat Intake and Diet Quality Among US Adults, 1999–2016." *JAMA* 322, no. 12 (September 2019): 1178–87. doi:10.1001/jama.2019.13771.

Tan, Yi, Zongke Wei, Jiaoliu Chen, Junli An, Manling Li, Liuyun Zhou, Yanhua Men, and Shan Zhao. "Save Your Gut Save Your Age: The Role of the Microbiome in Stem Cell Ageing," *Journal of Cellular and Molecular Medicine* 23, no. 8 (August 2019): 4866–75. doi:10.1111/jcmm.14373.

United States Food and Drug Administration. "FDA Warns About Stem Cell Therapies," last accessed August 9, 2019, https://www.fda.gov/consumers/consumer-updates/fda-warns-about-stem-cell-therapies?utm_campaign=11.16.17%20stem%20cell%20therapies&utm_medium=email&utm_source=Eloqua.

United States Food and Drug Administration. "Therapeutic Cloning and Genome Modification," last accessed August 6, 2019, https://www.fda.gov/vaccines-blood-biologics/cellular-gene-therapy-products/therapeutic-cloning-and-genome-modification.

Wing, Rena R, and Suzanne Phelan. "Long-Term Weight Loss Maintenance," *The American Journal of Clinical Nutrition* 82, no. 1 (July 1, 2005): 222S–225S. doi:10.1093/ajcn/82.1.222S.

INDEX

digestive system. *See also*
    gastrointestinal (GI) tract
    liver & intestines, fasting and,
        96
Dirty Dozen list, 115–116
DIY biology. *See* biohacking
drinking water, 50–52
dysbiosis, 101, 105

E

Eat Stop Eat, 92
elimination diets, 138
embryonic stem cells, 9
empowering readers, 155–156
empty calories, 38
energizing readers, 155–156
enlightening readers, 155–156
enterocytes. *See* absorptive cells
enteroendocrine cells, 20
environment, biohacking, 137–138
environmental toxins, 113
epidermal stem cells, 20
epigenetic mark, 17
epithelial stem cells, 19–20
ethical considerations, 15–16
Evolutionary theory, 78
exercise, 81–82, 125
extra-virgin olive oil (EVOO), 42

F

fasting
    alternate-day, 92
    and prolonged water fasting,
        160–161
    intermittent, 92
    as intervention, 151, 153–154
    long-term, 96–98
    mechanisms behind, 87–91

prolonged, 91
regimens, 86–87
stem cells, 112–113
styles of, 91–92
systemic benefits of, 96
fasting-mimicking diets (FMDs),
    93–94, 145–150
    working of, 95
fats, 40–42
    stem cells
        foods to exclude or reduce,
            122–123
        healthy, 121
fat-soluble vitamins, 46–47
fetal stem cells, 13
fish, 118
follicular stem cells, 20
Food for Young Children, 54
Food Guide Pyramid, 56
food-preparation methods,
    123–124
4-7-8 method, 126–127
Friedman School of Nutrition
    Science and Policy, 53
fruits, 120
functional nutrition, 2–4

G

gastrointestinal (GI) tract, 61–62,
    101
ghrelin, 71
glaucoma, 14
glucagon, 73
gluconeogenesis, 87
goblet cells, 19
good manufacturing practices
    (GMPs), 134
graft-versus-cancer effect, 24

graft-versus-host disease (GVHD), 24

gut lining, 104–105

H

Hassle-Free Guide to a Better Diet, 55

healthy gut, 99–111

heart stem cells, 10

heart/cardiovascular system, fasting and, 96

hematopoietic stem cells (HSCs), 18

herbs/spices, 121

Hippocrates, 61, 102

Hippocratic Oath, 61

HIV-associated dementia, 14

homeostasis, 60–61

How to Select Foods, 54

human body, 60–61
    as fine-tuned machine, 62–63
    gastrointestinal tract command center, 61–62

human embryonic stem cells, 11

hunger
    calorie, 63–65
    calories-in-calories-out, 72–74
    Cunningham Formula, 66–69
    factors influencing BMR, 65
    human body, 60–61
        as fine-tuned machine, 62–63
        gastrointestinal tract command center, 61–62
    Katch-McArdle Formula, 66
    losing, 69–72
    Mifflin-St Jeor Equation, 66

    Original Harris-Benedict Equation, 66
    Revised Harris-Benedict Equation, 66

Huntington's chorea, 14

hydration, 126

I

immune health, 101–111

increased intestinal permeability, 104

induced pluripotent stem cells (iPSCs), 11, 16

inflammation, 112–113

insulin, 72–73

intermittent fasting (IF), 92, 138, 162

iodine, 50

iron, 48–49

K

Katch-McArdle Formula, 66
    short-term, 151

L

Lancaster County Physician, 128

leaky gut syndrome, 104–105, 106

leptin, 71–72

light therapy, 137–138

L-Nutra, 93

Longevity Diet, The, 93

long-term fasting, 96–98

long-term weight-loss success, 68

low-quality foods, 114–117

M

macrominerals, 47–48

macronutrients. *See also specific macronutrients*
    carbohydrates, 37–39

T

U

V

W

Z

ACKNOWLEDGMENTS

First, I would like to thank my family and friends for their enduring love and support, and for understanding the time commitment that this endeavor required on top of my already-overextended schedule. This would not have been possible without their support (and our furbabies, who often sat by my side for hours while I was at the computer researching and writing).

To my two dietetic student researchers, Caitlyn Kambouroglos and Brooke Garman: May you continue to be inspired to seek the root causes impeding optimal health in your clients.

To my DIFM and MUIH families: Each of you provide me with daily inspiration to continue working hard toward the day that all nutritionists practice through an integrative and functional lens. I am blessed to have you in my life.

To Drs. Anton, Brandhorst, and Yilmaz: Thank you for sharing your time, knowledge, and expertise with me. Your work is changing lives, and I'm grateful for all you do.

Lastly, I'd like to thank the team at Ulysses Press. It was an honor and a pleasure to work with you.

ABOUT THE AUTHOR

Dana M. Elia, DCN-c, MS, RDN, LDN, FAND is an integrative and functional dietitian-nutritionist with close to 25 years of experience. Originally from New Jersey, Dana relocated to Lancaster, Pennsylvania, in 2001. She is the owner of Fusion Integrative Health and Wellness, LLC, which recently received the 2019 Best of Lancaster award in the nutritionist category. Dana is also an adjunct faculty member at the Pennsylvania College of Health Sciences. An active member of her community, Dana serves on the executive committee of Dietitians in Integrative and Functional Medicine, where she holds the chair position and previously served as chair-elect, treasurer, and member services chair.

Dana has recently been chosen to be a part of a select group of expert nutrigenomic providers to roll out the US launch of 3x4 Genetics and will also be serving as a mentor to other providers.

Dana previously served on the executive committees for the Lancaster Area Celiac Support Group and the Lancaster Chapter of the American Holistic Nurses Association. As a recognized leader in integrative and functional nutrition, Dana has provided content reviews for projects such as the fifth edition of the *Academy of Nutrition and Dietetics Complete Food and Nutrition Guide*. She regularly speaks to both lay and professional audiences, and has been featured in, or authored, numerous articles for *Natural Awakenings Magazine* and *LNP*.

Dana's dedication and fervor for the power within food as medicine stems from her own personal journey with autoimmune disease and a rare form of sarcoma. As a survivor and warrior for rare disease advocacy, Dana was chosen in 2017 as one of four survivors to be featured in videos with the Fox Chase Cancer Center and Temple University.

With a passion for ongoing education and a drive to give her patients the best level of care, Dana is currently finishing her doctorate in clinical functional nutrition (DCN) through the Maryland University of Integrative Health, where in 2019 she was awarded the Student Research Poster Award. In her free time, she loves hiking, camping, kayaking, scuba diving, traveling with her husband James and family, or spoiling her rescued fur-babies, Champ, Jasper, and George.